Unity and Multiplicity

Multilevel Consciousness of Self in Hypnosis, Psychiatric Disorder and Mental Health

Unity and Multiplicity

Multilevel Consciousness of Self in Hypnosis, Psychiatric Disorder and Mental Health

by

JOHN O. BEAHRS, M.D., A.B.M.H.

BRUNNER/MAZEL, *Publishers* • New York

Original graphics for figures by Matthew Hastie.

SECOND PRINTING

Library of Congress Cataloging in Publication Data

Beahrs, John O., 1940–
  Unity and multiplicity.

  Bibliography: p.
  Includes index.
  1. Multiple personality.   2. Dissociation
(Psychology)   3. Hypnotism—Therapeutic use.
4. Personality.   I. Title.   [DNLM: 1. Self
concept.   2. Hypnosis.   3. Dissociative
disorders.   4. Consciousness.   WM 173.6 B365u]
RC569.5.M8B47   616.85 ′236   81-38538
ISBN 0-87630-273-8   AACR2

Copyright © 1982 by John O. Beahrs

Published by

BRUNNER/MAZEL, INC.

19 Union Square

New York, New York 10003

MANUFACTURED IN THE UNITED STATES OF AMERICA

This book is dedicated to
MILTON H. ERICKSON, M. D.

From simple commonsense psychology, plus keen awareness of the need to communicate simultaneously at many levels, arose the vast armamentarium of elegant and imaginative techniques which are synonymous with the work of Milton H. Erickson. From an all pervasive integrity came his legendary flexibility, like branches from a well-rooted tree.

Modern clinical hypnosis, double-bind theory, and many forms of strategic and family therapies — all are outgrowths of his work.

The Master of Paradox, Milton H. Erickson exemplifies the creative force which is opening new vistas and leading psychotherapy into new dimensions which were hard to imagine only a few years ago.

We will long cherish his memory.

Acknowledgments

First, I would like to thank my many patients. They have courageously shared their struggles and faced what at times seemed like insurmountable obstacles to the joy of living. In addition, I owe much to the psychiatric staff of Western State Hospital and Puget Sound Hospital, Tacoma, Washington, for a setting where creative experimentation was not only permitted within a context of solid basics, but also encouraged.

Three colleagues deserve special mention for their help in clarifying the nuts and bolts of *Unity and Multiplicity*. Ernest R. Hilgard, in whose research laboratory I gained my first experience working with formal hypnosis, more recently formulated his neodissociation theory, which has provided much stimulus to my own thinking. Milton H. Erickson contributed information, guidance, and support at nearly all levels of my being during a very rich association. Most recently, John G. Watkins has provided generously of his time, energy, and support in reviewing manuscripts and giving critical feedback.

I would like to especially thank my mother, Virginia Oakley Beahrs, who not only did what is needed to ensure my own existence, but also devoted an intensive week's time to a massive editorial review

of the manuscript. Finally, my wife, Claudette, is herself a psychotherapist with a keen awareness of the importance of multiple consciousness to mental health. Her ability to resonate creatively with her
clients and share ideas at a high level is a continuing inspiration.

J.O.B.

Contents

Foreword

The concept that one might be a "multiplicity" rather than a "unity" is frightening. That there might lie within our self entities which we do not experience as "me" and over whose actions we may not have control strikes at the very heart of our self-concept. It threatens man's views of ethical responsibility. Moreover, if a single "person" cannot be completely equated with a single "body," if it is possible that we do not always know with whom we are dealing, then our entire system of jurisprudence is threatened.

The same fear of the uncontrollable, which in the past caused people to reject a Copernican concept of the universe, an evolutionary view of human development, and the existence of unconscious processes, impels us to deny the suggestion that each of us may be a multiplicity—not a single, unified self. Thus, diagnosticians avoid giving the label of multiple personality to a patient, even in the face of strong evidence, because they do not understand this condition and do not know how to treat it. Diagnoses such as schizophrenia or sociopathic personality, difficult as they are to treat, at least leave us on familiar ground. We think we know with what we are dealing. We do have some therapeutic approaches for the psychoses and legal methods of control for the sociopaths. But what do we do when we are confronted with two or more apparently different individuals existing within a single physical form?

In his ingenious therapeutic strategies, Milton Erickson exhibited a genuine awareness of the fact that individuals can be multiplicities as well as unities. He communicated with his patients at more than one level. Yet he did this almost as an unconscious art, not one which he formulated into an easily transmitted science.

Ernest Hilgard at Stanford University has demonstrated in his laboratory the existence of different cognitive structural systems indicating the presence of co-consciousness in relation to hearing and the perception of pain. And our own studies on ego states (J.G.W. & H.H.W.), as well as those by the author of this book, have shown quite clearly that dissociation is not simply an "either-or" phenomenon, a few strange individuals being "multiple personalities" and everybody else constructed as a "unity." Separateness and togetherness are relative, within individuals as well as between them. Syndromes of behavior and experience, both overt and covert, which cohere and are separated from one another by boundaries varying in permeability, are a fact of human personality organization, whether they are called "ego states," "hidden observers," "cognitive structural systems" or "multiple personalities."

The study of dissociation promises to bring a new perspective to the understanding of human personality and the treatment of its disorders. It is not enough for a behavior therapist to apply a reinforcement to an entire individual when it is a particular segment or ego state within that patient that needs the change. It is not sufficient for a global interpretation to be administered by an analyst to that body on the couch when a specific, child cognitive system within is the one exhibiting the transference. As therapists we need much greater sophistication concerning the interaction of an entire person with his/ her various facets of self if we are to do better than fire therapeutic shotguns in the generally right direction.

The study of dissociation, multiple personality, hidden observers and ego states opens the possibility of acquiring better maps of personality organization. These concepts, whether derived from theory, research or clinical observation, may also enable us to approach more intelligently the treatment of many other conditions in addition to the

classical dissociative disorders such as amnesias and multiple personalities. Some of our treatment and studies at the University of Montana have indicated that "ego-state therapy" can be applicable in
such nonpathologic, normal conditions as stopping smoking, weight
reduction and the improvement of study habits. We are learning that
individuals, like nations, have organized control segments, and that
consideration must be given to "state's rights," as well as to the "national welfare," if we are to help patients to organize their multiplicities into coherent, cooperative and well-functioning unities. That is
the thesis of this book.

John Beahrs is a practicing psychiatrist, sensitive therapist and
creative thinker. In this original work he, unlike the writers of most
clinical texts, is not content merely to describe the patients whom he
has treated, cite the relevant literature and demonstrate his therapeutic tactics. He has done all this, but he has also done much more.
From the multiplicity of observations, research reports, clinical data
and past theoretical concepts he has attempted to put together a
greater unity in man's view of life itself, man's relationship to himself,
his fellowmen, the universe and his God. This treatise is, therefore,
much more than a clinical cookbook on how to diagnose and treat
multiple personalities. Its author has wrestled mightily with the "six-
ty-four dollar" questions which have plagued humans from the first
realization of their own existence and their wonderment of how that
selfness came to be and how it is related to the great world about
them.

In multiple personalities we see the interaction of the "me" and the
"not-me." Our patients clearly demonstrate that "not me's" can be
carved out of segments of self which previously were "me," but which
with intelligent help can be induced to again experience "me-ness."
However, we can no longer be sure just at what point our "self" ceases
and an "it" begins. The study of dissociation brings a humble appreciation of just how fluid boundaries are and how our own "selves" relate
to, interact with and become a part of the greater world outside.

It is to Beahrs' credit that he has attempted to search out in his patients new conceptions of man's questions about existence. Accordingly, this treatise is a clinical work, insightful, sensitive and loaded
with practical suggestions for the psychotherapist, many of these most
ingenious and innovative. The mental health practitioner cannot

read it without finding exciting new vistas. Especially promising is his proposal of turning liabilities into assets, of converting a symptom into a skill.

This book is also a philosophical work. Logicians will appreciate how Beahrs has tried to make sense of his data through a rational approach, pulling together clinical observations with empirically-derived research findings toward newer and larger "unities." It is a book for the thinker, the philosopher, as well as for the treater. In his philosophical approach to the data, he forces his clinical readers to move beyond their therapeutic technology into the broader vistas of what their effort to better their patient's condition is all about. He impels practicing clinicians to become also contemplative theoreticians.

Finally, Beahrs has dared to strike out beyond the realm of research data, clinical observation and accepted personality theory into the area of religion. He rejects the thesis that "theology" has no place in clinical practice. In a truly religious (but nonsectarian) vein he affirms that our eyes must be upon the stars as well as on the ground, that man's understanding of his own self requires that he explore his relation to his God within this universe. In this respect he is an existentialist. He does not force upon us a pre-digested religion; he only stimulates us to share with him speculations about greater questions of being, of origins and of destinies.

The goals to which he aspires can never be fully attainable to man. But in his search for greater unity out of this multiplicity, Beahrs directs our gaze from the finiteness of self-segments within a fragmented patient to a oneness of mankind with his entire universe.

JOHN G. WATKINS, PH.D.
HELEN H. WATKINS, M.A.
University of Montana

Unity and Multiplicity

Multilevel Consciousness of Self in Hypnosis, Psychiatric Disorder and Mental Health

1

Simultaneous

Co-consciousness

The purpose, content and methods behind this book are summarized by the title—*Unity and Multiplicity: Multilevel Consciousness of Self in Hypnosis, Psychiatric Disorder and Mental Health.* First and foremost it is about *unity*, the essence of the human condition as we usually experience and describe it. The central issue is our selfhood, experienced as a type of unity in itself, even while it depends on having a place in and merging with a greater overall order of reality. It is about *multiplicity* to the extent that each of our individual "Self-s" is itself an "order of reality" within which other consciously experiencing "selves" have their *own* conscious experience and sense of selfhood, simultaneous with our own. We may indeed be true multiple personalities in a far more literal sense than the way the term is defined in the psychiatric nomenclature. *Simultaneous co-consciousness* existing within and perhaps even contributing to the essence of our "Cohesive Self" is the unifying theme of all my discussion, whether I am talking of research and clinical data which led me to this assumption, to its applications in psychiatry and the allied mental health professions, or to wider philosophical implications.

3

The body of data and experience leading to this study originally comes from and remains grounded in the phenomena of *hypnosis,* an area of personal and professional interest and expertise. Multilevel consciousness and communication are essential to the hypnotic process, even though we do not fully understand their essence. Of particular importance for clinical work is Hilgard's (1977) recent demonstration of intact ''hidden observers'' in even deeply hypnotized subjects; these hidden observers perceive differently from the hypnotized subject and have a consciousness which is, in a very real sense, their own. Freud's (1920) likening of hypnosis to love in both involving a loosening of ego boundaries and merging with what is beyond, but in a way which enhances one's sense of self, provides a balance to Hilgard's formulation by linking hypnosis to the issue of unity and multiplicity at all levels. In hypnosis both of these processes — existing as several selves and merging with what is outside the self — are positive; they enhance what we loosely term "mental health."

Another set of data and experience comes from my work as a practicing psychiatrist, especially from my work with a certain type of "difficult patient." For this type of patient, problems in his* sense of the unity and multiplicity of his selfhood describe, if not virtually define, his mental disorder. At one extreme is the multiple personality, within whom two or more "entities," each experiencing selfhood as if he were a whole person, vie with one another for control. At the other is the "symbiotic psychosis," where the person has such difficulty distinguishing "self" from "beyond" as to render reality-testing difficult. While one of these processes usually predominates, they are generally present simultaneously, as in hypnosis. Here the same processes which were seen as positive in the domain of hypnosis are seen as negative; they detract from what we call "mental health."

This leads to the central philsophical issue, which will be raised again and again throughout the book:

• *When is it useful or not useful to look upon an individual as a single unit, a "Cohesive Self"?*

---

*For convenience and readability, the male pronouns he, his, himself have been used throughout this book.

- *When is it useful or not useful to look upon any one as being con-stituted of many parts, each with an identity of his own?*
- *When is it more useful to see ourselves as a part of a greater whole?*

I use the term "useful" rather than "true" since all are true — simul-taneously and at all times. Molecules have their identity simultane-ously with the cells to which they contribute, these simultaneously with the human organism of which they are just a tiny part and the latter simultaneously with that which is yet beyond — families, nations and All That Is (Roberts, 1972). This awareness precludes judging our discussion primarily on truth value and unavoidably leads to a type of utilitarianism. The issue becomes: When does one perspective work and when not? And, when faced with the latter situation, are there things we can do to shift to the former, so that *what was once a symptom becomes a skill?*

In the seventy-plus years since Freud's pioneering work, psychiatric knowledge has increased by such leaps and bounds that the most re-cent compendia of psychiatric knowledge require multiple volumes. Psychoanalytic theories give us new understanding of how we think and feel and open many doors which formerly seemed shut. Perhaps the most important insight from psychoanalytic theory is that there is something going on beneath or beyond what we consciously experi-ence. Biological advances offer a path in other new directions. Com-plex even in its infancy, the science of psychobiology leads us to marvel at the seemingly perfect design of our bodies and brains. Studies in cross-cultural psychiatry give us still other insights as to what is unique to the nature of man, as opposed to characteristic of specific cultures. Efforts currently devoted to community mental health help us learn new things about the nature of social organiza-tions that will have a lasting impact on our attempts to shape our own destiny. The list is long. Yet, I cannot escape the feeling, despite the importance of our increasingly massive burden of knowledge, that something very basic is often overlooked. What is missing?

In our effort to work out all the complexities of observable reality, I believe that we often overlook the simple facts, which otherwise would be staring us in the face. There are directly observable facts of life known even to the ancients — empirical observations about our basic

biology, psychology, and spiritual needs — which are often overlooked
by mental health practitioners. Not only does it feel better to me, but
I also believe that it works better in helping troubled patients "get better," to keep things as simple as we can, even at the risk of being too
simple or simplistic. It is *too* simple, however, only if the rest of our
knowledge is ignored or the data contradicted, neither of which I am
suggesting that we do. There may be as much information in the simplicity of a Mozart sonata as in the most intricate of Wagner's operas;
a similar comparison may be even more relevant when it comes to
psychiatric theory. Ideally, the simple can encompass even more information than the complex, perhaps because of, rather than in spite
of, its simplicity. To search for simple unifying principles is one of the
major purposes of this book.

This presentation differs in several ways from many psychiatric
theories that deal with component parts of the psyche and their interaction. First, I do not propose *any* such formal theory of psychological
structure — in other words, no "Beahrsian psychodynamics." Instead,
I suggest that we use a simpler working model, an analogy rather than
a theory, which I refer to as a *conductor-orchestra model*. This applies in some way to any complex organization of energy; it is hardly
limited to the human mind-brain. Since this is far less specific than a
scientific theory, it may provide a unifying framework within which
specific theories fit — a "meta" theory perhaps; however, I prefer to
describe it as just a working model. Secondly, in applying this model I
prefer a strategic withdrawal from adherence to any of the well en-
trenched, established theories. I prefer to seek refuge in what I would
call simple, commonsense psychology, basically that which has been
known about human behavior and motivation throughout recorded
history. Third, in applying this model to clinical practice, when talking about any component part of a person's psyche, this part is not just
an abstract "mechanism"; it is, rather, seen as a *consciously experiencing being with which we can and must communicate.*

My favorite metaphor for understanding and working with human
behavior is to liken the human mind to a symphony orchestra. Like
the overall Self, the orchestra is a complex whole with a personality of
its own. Like any multicellular organism or social group, it is composed of many component parts or orchestra members, each with its own
sense of identity and unique personality, but all of which function

together in a coordinated cooperative endeavor to the advantage not only of the whole, but of all the parts. While the music is made entirely by the composite of parts, which transcends being a mere algebraic sum, it is held together and organized by the leadership of an executive, the conductor. Although he makes none of the actual music, the conductor is in charge — at one level a fundamental paradox, at another simple commonsense knowledge available to all of us.

The concept of the unconscious is as critical to my work as it is to Freud's (1916), though my concept is quite different from his. Hypnotherapists do not see the unconscious as a teeming cauldron of untamed fury almost crying for suppression so that society can survive, to be dealt with by a hierarchy of "defense" mechanisms. Rather, the unconscious is seen as the source of all life and growth. Being a repository of all our prior learning and experiences, it must clearly contain information far in excess of what is usually available to awareness. It is this collective of all our component parts which I liken to the orchestra, that which actually makes the music of life. The "conscious," ideally, correlates with the executive or conductor, an organizing force which must be in charge even while doing little of what is better done by the orchestra itself. Hypnotherapists often find that, contrary to the view of some psychoanalysts, the unconscious is more likely than the conscious to be cooperative, dependable, realistic, and workable. We therefore do our best to access this composite "unconscious" consciousness by all means available, while dealing with the conscious respectfully enough to preserve its pride, reinforce its need to be in charge and avoid unnecessary resistance.

For the functionality that we call "mental health" we need more than just the basics of mutual cooperation under an organizing leadership. Each part must know the role it best performs and do its best to fulfill it, not trying to usurp a role which is more appropriately lived by another part. Furthermore, all parts must treat one another with *respect*. The triad of 1) coordinated cooperative function among parts or levels of consciousness, 2) adherence of each to its most appropriate role, and 3) mutual respect is necessary not only for healthy living but also for effective psychotherapy.

Simple "commonsense psychology" assumes that people do what makes them feel good and what makes those they care about feel good and then reflects back upon themselves. People do what they perceive will fulfill goals which they have set for themselves; when these are lacking, they do their best to define their goals or a sense of direction in life. People do what they perceive is in accord with or furthering their basic values and beliefs about what is important to life. People like to have fun. They also like to discipline themselves when they perceive that this will be to some later advantage. People do what enhances their sense of pride in themselves and their sense of having some place in the order of reality. While people like to feel safe, they also seek a certain amount of adventure and like to rise to the challenges of life. People enjoy loving and being loved. People enjoy a certain amount of competitive aggression. People feel better when they can identify with and have faith in something beyond themselves.

This is indeed simple. Why do so many human beings, especially those we call "psychiatric patients," seem to violate these commonsense tenets of life and to strive toward negative outcomes even while proclaiming that they are not happy with life and would like things to be different? This issue has led to extensive psychiatric theorizing. My own way of dealing with it is simply to return to the basic premise underlying this whole work—that consciousness and behavior within a human organism are occurring simultaneously at more than one level. What most of us term healthy living requires that the simple commonsense psychologies of all the different levels, parts or aspects of a personality coordinate with one another to mutual advantage.

If we assume that in some sense there is more than "just one of us" in all people, the apparent contradictions resolve. If any *part* follows the tenets of commonsense psychology but two or more parts are either out of synchrony or at open odds with one another, the issue is clarified. A negative outcome, or unhappiness might ensue more from default than from choice, if the parts of an individual are sufficiently discordant and equally matched so as to paralyze the overall self's power for action. Likewise, one part might get his way, but the "he" who gets his way is not the same "entity" as the consciously experiencing "self." Thinking in this manner, the possibilities are virtually limitless and hardly require our subscribing to any one detailed theory of behavior.

Ericksonian treatment methods might appear unusual, if not bizarre, because communication is directed to a part or an aspect of consciousness not experienced as conscious by the overall self and not evident to most observers. Most of us respond primarily to the most overt levels of words and behavior. When we respond to what is or seems hidden, this appears bizarre—bizarre but appropriate, and therefore effective.

Symphony orchestras can be organized in many different ways. Some have large string sections; others have small string sections. Some have large brass sections; others nonexistent brass sections. In some orchestras the conductor is an entirely separate agency making none of the music; in other groups, especially small ensembles, the conductor will also be playing one of the instruments, like the first violin. In some orchestral styles, the different sections are discrete and alternate, while in others all parts function together as an integrated whole.

Most detailed psychiatric theories could be likened to one particular way in which an orchestra might be organized. To the extent that this is appropriate to all human minds, such theory would prove relevant. I am not convinced that this is the case, however, and suspect that the human mind-brain can be organized in at least as many ways as orchestras and chamber ensembles. My clinical experience suggests that one particular psychiatric framework may work better with one person and not another, that a different model works better with another, and that we cannot predict which will work in any instance on the basis of psychiatric diagnosis. I have yet to find an established rule of behavior which doesn't appear to have exceptions. I suspect that our brains permit us to organize our mental life in at least as many ways as societies can be governed. This is no more than a restatement of what has always been known—that each human being is unique, even while sharing the essence of humanness with everyone else. The clinical relevance of this assumption is that it is best to keep our eyes and ears open to whatever aspects and parts of an individual we can observe, without any preconceived ideas of how they "should" or must be and interact. Contacting each part of the individual in a respectful manner, we can find out what each wants and believes and from this how things are going wrong. Just as in international diplomacy, progress is more likely to result if the unique needs of all parts are given adequate attention and respect. The ability to do this effectively at the intrapsychic level is required for a good hypnotherapist and is a valuable asset for all psychotherapists.

An increasingly large body of hard scientific data, so far unexplained, convincingly supports this basic position. This is the collection of mental phenomena loosely termed "hypnosis." While the body
of information about hypnosis is growing by leaps and bounds, as with
all science, no formal theory about hypnosis has even begun to survive
the snares of its own internal contradictions. I do not make any pretense of attempting to correct this situation. I do not understand hypnosis and do not know of anyone who does, but I hope that my experience in working with it will help me to clarify some thoughts about
why this strange state of affairs persists — and perhaps must.

The study of hypnosis unavoidably forces us to examine the many
time-worn philosophical dilemmas usually ignored by our profession.
The nature of objective and subjective "reality," subject versus object,
free will versus determinism, good and evil, faith and belief, and the
nature and limits of human knowledge — these are only but a representative sample. In the concluding essay and epilogue of my earlier
book, *That Which Is* (1977a), I discussed the importance of these
issues to mental health. While the current book is more clinical than
philosophical, the very focus of attention is such that the issues pop up
again and again, to my delight.

Interestingly, the primary data of clinical relevance emerging from
the study of hypnosis concern co-consciousness. While not explaining
this phenomenon, hypnotic data at least demonstrate the existence of
simultaneous multilevel consciousness in mentally healthy individuals. When we are treating a patient where this is a problem — a
multiple personality, for example — the philosophical dilemmas just
referred to appear again, and at a level much closer to where we all
live. It is impossible to treat a multiple personality successfully
without facing all of these issues and more, in a way which is unique to
each patient. Perhaps this is why multiple personality, like hypnosis,
is so fascinating to the lay public. It may also shed some light on why it
is so assiduously avoided by the mental health profession at large. As
professionals we have been trained to avoid anything like "theology"
or philosophy, for at least two reasons: 1) to respect a patient's right to
his own value system, and 2) to not extend our specialty beyond its
scientific bounds where it would then necessarily lose its preciseness
and become "fuzzy." Yet, even the most meticulous scientific study of
hypnosis and multiple personality forces us to that very point!

When I find that for any seemingly true belief its opposite can be argued just as convincingly and when my experience suggests that the area of inquiry where this most often occurs is that which is most important in understanding what life is all about, I become much less enthusiastic about working out the type of precise, detailed thinking necessary for a psychiatric theory. When exceptions become as important as the rules, the theory becomes much less satisfying and it becomes more comfortable to withdraw to what is more a basic faith than a belief: *all that is simply is*. While I remain firm in my belief and faith in a primary reality or "that which is," I am equally aware that we actually know only the experience of ourselves, seeing that which is outside of us only from the limits of an external observer. Even in physics, that most precise of all sciences, Feynman, Leighton and Sands (1963) state that each piece, or part, of the whole of nature is always merely an approximation to the complete truth.

Belief systems can be likened to two-dimensional photographs of a three-dimensional object. If adequate, a photo taken from one perspective is as true as another, though it may seem totally different. Each is true, but only part of the story. The implication is that there is one primary *all that is,* but a potentially infinite number of adequate, equally true and different ways in which it can be perceived and understood. Many may appear to contradict one another and these paradoxes may not all be capable of clear solution. Perhaps the best we can do is accept the seemingly polar opposites and paradoxical elements in all that is, recognizing that we cannot always distinguish boundaries between one and the other or be entirely clear and precise when only one polarity applies. The *whys* of such opposites as proton and anti-proton, male and female, a free choice and something which just happens, good and evil, we do not understand fully — we just *observe* these distinctions. While we can accumulate more data, we don't know the whys but must accept many of these polar opposites as *givens* with which we must work.

ORGANIZATION OF THIS BOOK

The plan for organizing this book now emerges. The first order of business is to take a close look at that large body of scientific data, hypnosis, which so inconveniently clogs up the machinery of our most refined theories. I will summarize the hypnotic data and delineate the issues for further inquiry which emerge. Multilevel consciousness and questions about volition and executive control are those of most relevance to the practicing clinician. After having clarified the status of these, I will share come clinical case material showing their relevance first to everyday life and then to what we call "psychopathology." Much of the latter will be seen as similar to autohypnosis, occurring spontaneously out of the individual's executive control and in a manner to his detriment. Knowing the value of autohypnotic skill, the pragmatic question is the extent to which we might be able to bypass traditional treatment methods, using instead hypnotic techniques with what is already a type of hypnosis to help him regain control, so that what was once a symptom becomes a skill.

Dissociative disorders, with multiple personality at the extreme end of a continuum, present a specialized form of multiple consciousness. These are examined in detail. Disorders at the other end of the spectrum, where the self merges with beyond in a type of symbiosis, receive somewhat less attention—not for lack of importance, but because they are more difficult to describe within the structure of our language. I will again share clinical material which illustrates treatment dilemmas which are raised.

The facets of these various dilemmas are discussed as they come up. For example, "possession" by what appears to be a demon, as well as other types of persecutory part-selves seen in clinical practice, force us to take a closer look at the problem of evil and its role in human life, one which is often paradoxical.

Another dilemma is the extent to which a psychotherapist can or should be like a new and better parent. The evidence of ever-present, adequately perceiving hidden observers in even the most disturbed borderline personalities suggests a drastic revision of the psychoanalytic method, without necessarily violating any of its theory. What formerly could be accomplished only by working through the transference may be more effectively and economically done by simply accessing, working with, and giving power for action to the hidden observer—which sees the analyst accurately whatever the state of transference at the overt level. Expansive syndromes, when selfhood goes beyond its usual boundaries, force us to take a critical look at phenomena usually termed "occult"; these challenge the exclusiveness of our current theories, even in physics. Perhaps most important clinically is the working observation that whenever we are talking about a component of the psyche, this part is not just an abstract "mechanism" used to help us organize our thoughts. It is an *actually experiencing being* which we can contact and communicate with and with which we *must* communicate respectfully if we are to effectively fulfill our responsibilities as psychotherapists.

The issues which emerge blend in a fine continuum with the experience of everyday life. In a very real sense we are all multiple personalities, and we also have some element of symbiotic psychosis. What is relevant to these syndromes is then relevant to all of us. If these entities raise unanswerable philosophical issues, we must now raise them for each and all of us. In the "Epilogue: Beyond Psychiatry," I will point towards implications of the unity and multiplicity approach to aspects of human life usually considered beyond the scope of our profession. Not the least of these is the need to find strength and rootedness in a basic faith and integrity which, paradoxically, can increase our power for both action and intellect, despite the increased awareness of the limitations inherent in any of our beliefs and theoretical systems.

2

Hypnosis and Trance—Posing Some Issues

Considering that nobody truly understands hypnosis, that domain of mental life holding such unique fascination in so many ways, the degree to which hypnotherapists share at least some consensus about how to employ it productively in the therapeutic process is remarkable. As a psychiatric subspecialty, hypnosis differs from others like psychoanalysis or transactional analysis (T.A.) in being not a theory but a collection of mental phenomena. Although we do not understand such behaviors and experiences, we must deal with them whatever our theoretical orientation. Nowhere in psychotherapy have I found a more striking example of the gulf between theory and practice in mental health. For this reason alone, hypnotherapists, whatever their original background, acquire an increasingly pragmatic orientation in their work.

Three dimensions of mental function — volitional, perceptual and cognitive — best define what is usually referred to as hypnotic, as illustrated on Figure 1. I will open the discussion by posing a representative question from each continuum of mental function; these questions raise familiar issues which are far from amenable to scientific explanation.

14

Figure 1
Three-factor Definition of Hypnosis

"Hypnotic" refers to phenomena relatively toward the righthand end of *three continua* of mental function.

Non-hypnotic		Hypnotic
Voluntary, Free choice, "I *do* it"	Volitional ___ Continuum	Involuntary, Spontaneous, "Just happens"
Structured perception of reality—out there	Perceptual ___ Continuum	*Fluidity* of perception, Vivid imagination, perceived imaginings, Possible distortions in all sense modalities
Secondary process, Reality logic	Cognitive ___ Continuum	Primary and tertiary processes, magical, symbolic, pictorial thinking, "Regression" in service of ego

1) Volitional: What distinguishes an individual intentionally lifting his hand with a full sense of free choice from one who experiences it as "just lifting," as though of its own accord? The distinction between voluntary and involuntary behavior and experience exemplifies the age-old free will versus determinism controversy in its psychiatric and everyday life contexts.

2) Perceptual: What differentiates one who observes the scene actually before him from one who, though fully awake with his eyes open, visualizes himself instead canoeing on a Minnesota lake, delighting in the shimmer of the birches, the ripple of the water, and perhaps a bird or two? I believe if we can ever explain how this hallucinatory experience differs from the simple imagining of such a scene, we will not only understand the distinction between our usual consciousness and the hypnotic state but will know vastly more about the human mind.

3) Cognitive: What separates ordinary thinking, productive but plodding, from sudden flashes of insight? For example, after struggling ineffectually to solve some crucial life dilemma, one may in the end surrender conscious will to something beyond himself—God,

the unconscious, or whatever — generating a profoundly moving experience. Inexplicably finding himself relaxing, he can enjoy passing thoughts and visual images, perhaps even a dream, and shortly thereafter discover that the seemingly insoluble problem has apparently solved itself — what had appeared impossible is now obvious. Only this third area of mental functioning is even remotely within the realm of what can be explained by current psychodynamic theory.

In Figure 1 these three dimensions are depicted separately, what is termed hypnotic appearing on the right hand end of each continuum. The first dimension, that of voluntary versus involuntary function, is one I posed as a major issue in *That Which Is* (1977a). Usual waking or non-hypnotic behavior is at the voluntary pole; we experience our actions as self-directed or chosen. While the voluntary dimension is rarely if ever completely absent in hypnosis, most subjects report an increase in automaticity in their behavior during what they call trance. A subject may experience her arm to be light as a feather, lifting up towards her face as if it "just happens," without any choice or voluntary effort. She might similarly feel her arm to be stiff and rigid and be unable to bend it no matter how hard she tries.

These are termed "motor phenomena" in the hypnotic literature (Hilgard, 1968); a "good" subject is one who responds to most suggestions with a hypnotic-like response. That the voluntary component of this behavior is beyond awareness may lead to the illusory aura of magic, which, unfortunately, too often surrounds hypnosis. To avoid misunderstanding, however, I must point out that emphasizing the involuntary nature of hypnotic behavior can be clinically misleading, since clinical hypnosis involving autohypnosis is one of the most potent ways of helping a patient achieve more voluntary control, a paradox that may be resolved to some degree by the conductor-orchestra analogy underlying this book.

The second continuum of mental function is perceptual. The polarity characterizing usual waking or non-hypnotic behavior is structured perception — perception as we usually experience it, with our percepts corresponding roughly to actually existing entities "out there" perceivable by others as well. At the pole I call "hypnotic" is fluidity of perception or perceived imaginings. During hypnosis, virtually all manner of perceptual distortion is possible. One minute of time may be experienced as only a second or two or as a month or a year. One may perceive an imagined scene as vividly as if it were actually there (positive hallucination), or may fail to see something squarely in the visual field (negative hallucination).

A variant of negative hallucination useful to doctors and dentists is hypnotic analgesia. A hypnotic subject may be able to tolerate not only such usually painful procedures as dental reconstruction or childbirth, but also major surgery.

A third continuum concerns the level of cognition. At the usual non-hypnotic pole, thinking is dominated by the reality principle or secondary process. While secondary process rarely vanishes totally during hypnosis, there is a relative preponderance of a more primitive type of thinking usually referred to as primary process because it develops much earlier in life than reality-testing. Magical thinking—concepts linked together by a common wish or emotional drive rather than by a common principle or fact—is characteristic of this. An unsophisticated hypnotic subject may even consider his responses as actually caused by the hypnotist in a quasi-magical way, failing to experience his own role consciously. Another subject may think in a pictorial and symbolic manner, with vivid visual images displaying the same primitive modes of logic, such as condensation and displacement, found in the dream work of Freud (1900). Or images may resemble more closely the symbols of Jung (1964), amenable to a more direct translation from the primary to secondary process language. The waking pole is characterized by verbal or digital language, with signs (words) bearing no physical resemblance to that which they denote. The hypnotic pole is more symbolic or analogical, with pictorial images in sense modalities that do resemble their data.

That implied hypnotic regression is actually "in the service of the ego" (Gill and Brenman, 1959) and usually under control of reality-testing, even when supplied by a hypnotist, suggests a major difference from the pure primary process found in some schizophrenias. In his study of the creative process, Arieti (1976) coined the term "tertiary process" to denote a level of cognition in which secondary and primary process are combined and integrated. The mind now has the greater flexibility and expansiveness of the deeper levels along with the protective supervision of reality-testing—the best of both worlds. Arieti's use of the word tertiary conveys his belief that this type of regression in the service of the ego actually constitutes an advance to a potentially higher level than pure reality-testing itself, a belief with which I fully concur.

In hypnosis, when reality-testing seems missing, it is not gone but only hidden, as discussed below in connection with research on hidden observers. The clinical implications of this lead to a striking new way of looking at psychiatric problems which is one of the central themes of this book. When some act is performed without being experienced by the conscious self as voluntary, it is often said to have been done by the unconscious. Yet what appears "unconscious" to the self proper may actually have been a conscious choice of one of its parts, illustrating the multiplicity inherent in the experience of selfhood.

Hypnosis is simply experience and behavior relatively toward the righthand end of each or all of these three continua of mental function — automaticity of action, fluidity of perception and primary or tertiary process thinking. This definition in itself suggests nothing about the point where one must arbitrarily indicate whether or not something is hypnotic when the boundaries are not distinct. As defined, all hypnotic behavior is waking behavior but not all waking behavior is hypnotic. Hypnosis is a differentiated type of waking state, then, but not always easy to define as an altered state of consciousness. To do this in any but an arbitrary manner would require a reliable, observable separation from the altered state and the baseline consciousness. With hypnosis, this is possible for some individuals, but not for others.

Trance denotes hypnotic states when they occur with discontinuity from non-hypnotic or different types of trance states. This is illustrated in Figures 2 and 3, using a method for distinguishing altered states of consciousness suggested by Tart (1975). Limited by the two-dimensional world of the printed page, these graphs depict only the first two continua of Figure 1 as the coordinates, leaving the reader to imagine that the third would be another coordinate perpendicular to the two on the page. For the present, we can assume that consciousness at any moment in time can be represented by a point at any spot on the graph, with different points on it representing the subject's consciousness at different times. Clusters of points then depict an individual's state of consciousness over a representative, extended

Figure 2

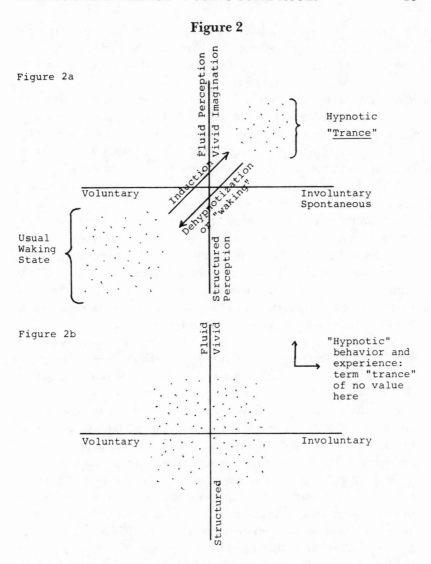

period of time. Points in the lower left quadrant refer to non-hypnotic consciousness as defined earlier, with voluntary action and structured perception. Those in the upper right are clearly hypnotic.

Figure 2a and 2b refer to different persons. The one portrayed by Figure 2a is an individual most of whose waking experience occurs in two clusters of consciousness, one hypnotic and the other not, with few points in the transitional area between. For this person, there is sufficient discontinuity between his hypnotic and non-hypnotic consciousness so that he would likely experience them as separate states of consciousness. Hypnosis, when it occurs as a separate state of consciousness, is termed trance. To get from the non-hypnotic to the trance state requires an induction passing through a transitional zone where there are few, if any, points of consciousness. The reverse, often termed "waking," is better referred to as dehypnotization, since all hypnotic behavior is waking in the most absolute sense.

While the individual portrayed in Figure 2b may have even more capacity for hypnotic experience than Mr. 2a, it is not meaningful for him to talk of trance as a separate state. Since there is no discontinuity or transitional zone for this individual, he functions more in an extended and flexible waking mode which encompasses the hypnotic. This is not a trance. Trance as a special state can be said to have relevance only if hypnotic behaviors are discontinuous from the rest of the subject's waking state. Both Mr. 2a and 2b experience hypnosis, but only in the former is trance felt to be a separate state.

Several unresolved issues in hypnosis can be put in relief by extending Tart's method to three more hypothetical cases, depicted in Figure 3. Mr. 3a is an individual whose behavior is always hypnotic—he is probably in deep trouble. Lacking structured perception and reality-testing, as well as behavior control, he is most likely a chronic psychotic. I believe that this constellation is only approached by the most severely disturbed schizophrenics, who probably suffer biological derangements far beyond the scope of this inquiry. Certain patients might superficially resemble Mr. 3a, however, where the needed non-hypnotic dimension is not *missing* but only *hidden*. In this case, we must ask: If and when there is a hidden observer, can it be accessed and empowered so that we can expeditiously have an integrated person? When this is possible, as in many borderline patients and multiple personalities, and how this can be achieved will be discussed in Chapters 5 and 6 on Dissociative Disorder.

Figure 3b illustrates an individual usually termed non-hypnotizable. Whether individuals incapable of hypnotic experience actually exist, or whether they are those with such discontinuity that it is hard to move from one state to another is a moot question for now, though it does illustrate questions about hypnotizability.

Figure 3

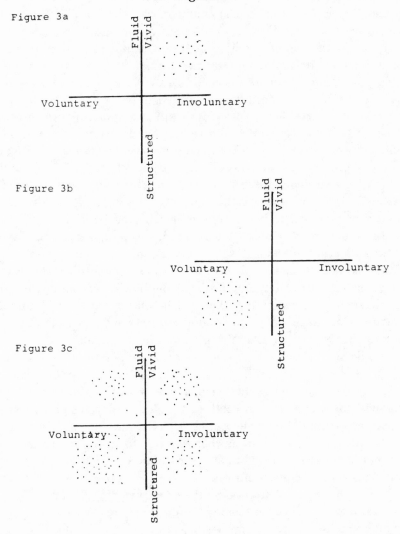

Figure 3a

Figure 3b

Figure 3c

More intriguing are possibilities inherent in Figure 3c. Perhaps there might be a cluster of points (state of consciousness) on the lower right in which most behavior is experienced as involuntary or spontaneous, though perception and imagination are little different from usual. This would correspond to an individual who responds to motor

challenge suggestions in a hypnotic induction, but is unable to experience cognitive effects such as hallucinations or time distortion. At
the upper left, an individual would be in a state in which he can experience all manner of cognitive distortion, hallucination, age regression, hypnotic dreaming and the like, but always with a sense of full
voluntary control, able to back this up by not responding to motor
suggestions like hand levitation or arm rigidity.

In point of fact, both types of individuals abound in both clinical
practice and research studies. There is no reason to preclude the possibility that there might be different clusters of points (different types of
trances) even in the same individual. Indeed, Barber (1975) has said
that "if you are going to talk about 'trance' to begin with, why talk
about THE trance? Maybe there are two, three, or even an infinite
number of types of trance" — a point worth consideration.

In concluding this initial step in organizing our conception of hypnosis and its implications, I want to clarify one basic point. These definitions are definitions and only that; they *explain* nothing. If they fit
common usage concisely and flexibly enough to be acceptable to most
clinicians and investigators, they will be of value in formulating a
common language, one I will develop throughout this book in clarifying the issues of unity and multiplicity in mental health.

While theoretical and methodological problems in hypnosis research are manifold, I will focus attention on only three. First is the
controversy concerning whether or not it is meaningful to consider
hypnosis or trance as a "special state." Not only is this dispute fascinating in itself, but it illustrates perfectly the limitations of any
theoretical system — that even when followed to an apparently logical
conclusion, it seems to end in absurdity. There are certain things we
may never fully explain but must live with and use as basic givens.

My second focus of attention is the issue of what we mean by "hypnotizability," meriting just enough discussion here to shed additional
light on the type of person for whom a clinical hypnosis model is most
relevant.

Third but most critical to the purpose of this entire inquiry is recent
research on hidden observers which poses the problem of defining dissociation so that it is not simply a manifestation of severe psychopathology but also essential to mental health, as exemplified in the hypnotic dimension. Only then can a single process appear both healthy and

pathological, opening the door to my clinical theme — the significance of taking charge of whatever is going on without necessarily changing its basic nature, so that what was once a symptom becomes a skill.

THE SPECIAL STATE CONTROVERSY—A/NOT-A ABSURDITY

In addition to being a subspeciality without a theory, hypnosis occupies another unique place in psychiatry and psychology. Like such potent issues as God, good/evil, freedom, and even psychiatry's multiple personality, hypnosis has believers ranged against non-believers concerning its very existence. Controversies of this sort, that allow a clear-cut stance either for or against a certain position regardless of the degree of actual knowledge on the subject, are few but of great importance. That these controversies involve specifically the concepts just mentioned is by no means accidental, as explained below. Indeed, in attempting to abstract key issues in the debate over whether or not there are really such things as hypnosis or trance, I find that at some level they implicate questions concerning God, good and evil, freedom, and multiple personalities.

On the surface the reader might share my own bewilderment as to why the existence of hypnosis is at issue, since its terms are definable as something to which we can all relate, whether or not we lay claim to substantial explanatory value. Nobody who has witnessed hypnotic behavior or enjoyed hypnotic experience can deny the occurrence of something profound and the need for adequate words with which to discuss it.

The underlying problem is, however, that if we cannot define any clear line of demarcation between hypnosis and nonhypnosis (what I here call A and Not-A), how can the distinction have pragmatic or scientific value? In contemporary debate, Barber (1972) has become the foremost spokesman for the Not-A or skeptical position concerning hypnosis; similar and other reservations are also raised by Sarbin and Coe (1972).

The first objection to trance as a special state is methodological in nature and involves the principle of parsimony, termed "Occam's Razor" by physicists. This principle states that if two or more theoretical constructs are equally able to explain certain data, that one is pre-

ferable which postulates the fewest entities or constructs capable of
encompassing the known data.

A second objection of the skeptical theorist to the concepts of hypnosis and trance is circularity. Observing, for example, a man responding far more markedly to suggestion than he ordinarily would,
one might ask, "Why is this?" and receive the answer, "Because he is
in a hypnotic trance."

"How do you know he is in a hypnotic trance?"

"Because he is responding to hypnotic suggestion."

Sarbin and Coe (1972) term this a pseudo-explanation that explains nothing and may even obscure accurate analysis of the data. It
occurs to me that the pseudo-explanation problem may have been
one of Freud's reasons for abandoning hypnosis, since he had so con-
spicuous a personal need to explain everything; even now hypnosis is
close to inexplicable. Barber and others have shown that such trance-
like characteristics as blank stare, limp posture, literalness of response
and possibly even trance logic might be artifacts not actually necessary to hypnotic behavior but inadvertently introduced by attitudes
and expectancies.

Control variables in hypnosis research are another thorn in attempts to define a special state. Barber has demonstrated a similar effect following task motivation as well as hyperalertness suggestions,
the opposite of the old "you are getting sleepy" type of induction. Edmonston (1972) has found the same response to relaxation instructions as to hypnotic inductions. Hilgard (1968) converged with almost
all other researchers in awareness of the extent to which simple imagination may lead to hypnotic behavior. It is, therefore, well established that most hypnotic effects can also be achieved by task motivation, types of work with relaxation and skilled use of imagery.

But if the target behaviors are by definition those to which the concept of hypnosis is applied and all control variables lead to these very
behaviors, this seems logically equivalent to saying that each of these
controls is in itself a hypnotic induction — a point raised by numerous
investigators that seems irrefutable to me. Skeptics claim that since
what are termed "hypnotic effects" can occur as a result of events
common throughout all waking life, there is little meaning in the
word. Alternatively, we could say that if all antecedent events leading
to a particular response are inductions, virtually the entire realm of
human life is hypnotic.

Whether one supports hypnosis or not, we are trapped in a major paradox. Either all our waking experience is non-hypnotic or it is all hypnotic. In either case, attempts to separate hypnotic from non-hypnotic phenomena lead to logical absurdity, even though the original defining conditions seemed appropriate.

The same paradox arises in somewhat more sophisticated form in the theorizing of Sarbin and Coe (1972). With a complex series of philosophical arguments, they discuss the nature of a hypnotic hallucination. This is a counter-factual perception not corresponding to what is really there, though believed in with subjective credulity. The issue of what is counter-factual and yet accepted (or we could say experienced at a conscious level) leads these investigators directly to the question of what is conscious as opposed to unconscious. Their conclusion is that the unconscious has no meaning and can more accurately be redefined as "choosing to withhold." This is similar to what Roberts (1974) termed "conscious but ignored."

The word *choosing,* implying freedom or volition in the everyday sense of those words (Beahrs, 1977a), leads us into difficulty here. If we choose to withhold something (render it unconscious), that seems to imply that we can as easily choose to not withhold or to return it to consciousness. Unlike the unconscious of Freud (1916), which he explicitly defined as what one cannot bring to awareness by voluntary effort, the element of choice brings us closer to Freud's preconscious—simply what is available but not being thought about at that particular moment. If we adhere to that part of our methodology requiring compatibility with common usage in defining complex terms, then involuntary choice is an obvious contradiction.

This leads directly into perhaps the single most important issue arising from the study of hypnosis—the problem of volition or the distinction between free choice and involuntary behavior. What is volition? What is free will? The age-old struggle between free will and determinism still lives on in the fields of both hypnosis and psychotherapy, despite claims (Beahrs, 1977a) that the concept of free will depends on determinism and that both are equally valid. Those who emphasize either polarity at the expense of the other get themselves into the same difficulty as Sarbin and Coe in connection with the conscious/unconscious dichotomy or the problem of all behavior being either non-hypnotic or hypnotic.

Hard determinists, including many of the original psychoanalysts, assert that what we call free choice is merely a subjective experience of forces obeying the same laws as all matter-energy, the implication being that free choice is an illusion. The same clinicians may paradoxically use a concept of "unconscious purpose" to imply that behavior not consciously experienced as a choice—such as certain convenient accidents—may have been instigated by some part of the personality that did actually so choose, though not consciously. In other words, the concept of free choice is now used in an attempt to explain what is usually considered not free but determined behavior.

Where is the boundary? Roberts (1974) has gone to the extreme of surmising that all naturally occurring events, even a specific birth date, time, and place, are freely chosen. What does taking such liberties do to our common-usage sense of the word freedom?

The problem posed by the trance-as-special-state controversy clearly extends far beyond the bounds of what we usally consider the domain of hypnosis. Not only can we not separate hypnosis from non-hypnosis without logical absurdity, but the same dilemma applies to voluntary/involuntary behavior and the conscious/unconscious. Logic in many ways favors the skeptics when boundaries within any of these dichotomies blur to where separation appears meaningless.

"All That Is" must ultimately be one gigantic and infinite unity with no absolute boundaries. The paradox is that we perceive and experience the multiplicity as not only very real, but of critical importance. Sense of selfhood as well as perception of any finite entities even depends upon it. Perhaps some Buddhist mystics hit close to the truth when they maintain that one's basic being depends on acceptance of what boils down to a cosmic joke—that the separateness that gives people their unique identities is never actually there, though they still depend upon it.

In attempting to analyze the dilemma we are in relative to the special state controversy—whether concerning hypnotic versus non-hypnotic phenomena, voluntary/involuntary action, or some other debatable distinctions (A against Not-A)—I refer to the impasse as the A/Not-A Absurdity. Whether arguing that all is A or that all is not—even without violation of logic or of data from the defining conditions themselves—the distinctions lose relevance. Not only is it equally possible to be a believer or non-believer, but the whole thing becomes purely a matter of personal preference.

In hypnosis, the absurdity is that the original definitions of hypnotic and non-hypnotic referred to dimensions of human experience to which almost all could relate. Although the distinction between A and Not-A was meaningful at a level of pure experience, when carried to its logical conclusion, it lost meaning in open violation of the original observable distinctions.

The process leading to the absurdity involves defining A and Not-A in clear operational terms, followed by logical analysis of sound objective data and defining conditions—only to come to the conclusion that certain aspects of what was previously defined as Not-A are actually A and vice versa! Thus the original definitions become inappropriate, even though referring to clearly observable distinctions.

Searching for what these particularly sensitive areas of discourse have in common, not shared by less controversial areas of science and philosophy, I find three features (in a sense just different ways of saying the same thing):

1) Limits of any definition are arbitrary. With hypnotic or non-hypnotic behavior, even using the three-factor definition of hypnosis that I favor, the point of distinction could be decided upon by a vote as opposed to a scientific experiment.
2) A and Not-A are at poles of a continuum.
3) Boundaries between entities along the continuum are not clear and measurable.

Every human being has experienced the difference between a free act and something that simply happens. Since nobody denies that the distinction is both relevant and critical to defining roles and to healthy living, arguments between professionals of even similar persuasion as to whether an individual chose a particular action (responsibility) or whether it "just happened" (victim) show the difficulties in defining the boundary.

Boundary problems exemplified by the A/Not-A Absurdity lead simultaneously in two directions. First, this dilemma must apply to any finite belief or belief system which, carried to its ultimate conclusion, can lead to the same absurdity. Even an entity with boundaries as clear and measurable as those of a given chair, for example, is not absolute (cf. Appendix I). Any entity is an abstraction (Beahrs, 1977a).

The A/Not-A Absurdity is, then, not unique to the special issues at hand; rather, it is an aspect of any finite belief or concept. When the defining conditions are as clear and measurable as those of a chair, the problem is not manifest, for we are then within the limits of relevance of the construct, where it is useful. When boundaries become blurred, by pushing their limits we encounter the absurdity. Not that concepts are not useful; in fact they are necessary. The absurdity is simply an expression of their limits, beyond which the construct becomes not false, but irrelevant. Considered in this light, much of psychiatry's task can be seen not as arguing over which belief or theory is more valid, but in defining the limits of relevance for each. We can ask ourselves in which setting one framework is more functional and in which another would work better.

Another direction where the A/Not-A problem leads is the heart of unity and multiplicity. This is the voluntary/involuntary issue. The fact that we can simultaneously choose and not choose to perform some act suggests multiplicity or co-consciousness. It may not always be either-or—it may be either-and. Hypnosis is the classic paradox *par excellence,* in that a subject may choose to do something and not do it at the same time—lifting his hand voluntarily, for instance, in a hand levitation, yet experiencing it as if it just happens.

Who is the doer? Who the experiencer? These questions would seem nonsensical if we were to look upon a human mind as simply a cohesive whole, even one divided into component mechanisms. The dilemma begins to soften when we consider each individual as having not just one self but at least two, like the Self 1 and Self 2 of Gallwey (1974), which I have elaborated upon elsewhere (1977a, b).

Yet we are now faced by an unavoidable and somewhat disquieting new datum about consciousness. In normal human individuals, at least while hypnotized, there may be two personalities or more, each with his own consciousness, of which the other part(s) may or may not be aware. As we recognize that boundaries between hypnosis and the usual waking state are fuzzy, if present at all, there is the likelihood that *consciousness occurs simultaneously at different levels within any human mind.* What will be conscious for one level or part-self may be unconscious for another—hence the difficulty in defining the conscious and unconscious in absolute terms. Bearing in mind that boundaries may be flexible, it is not irrelevant to consider that we might have an even infinite number of part-selves, each contributing to a unique cohesive self. The rudimentary yet significant contribution of current hypnosis research to exploring this possibility is considered below in my discussion of hidden observers.

It is clear that the trance-as-special-state controversy remains unresolved. I would not be surprised if this condition persists as long as that of its counterpart, freedom versus determinism—possibly throughout all future as well as past recorded time. For myself, the only way to find comfort in the morass of contradictory theories and data is to recognize that all may be true in a sense or, as Barber (1977) has said, "all true but only part of the story." I personally find it meaningful to distinguish between hypnotic and non-hypnotic phenomena by definitions, though clearly aware that all human mental processes could be conceptualized as one or the other with equal accuracy. The question is not truth but utility; when is one way of looking at it more useful?

The same dilemma raises its head in the diagnosis and treatment of dissociative disorders, such as the multiple personality. That both definitions and boundaries are indistinct may offend clinicians who seek greater precision, at times myself included. Yet I find no way out other than conceding that among the givens of life with which we must live and work are certain paradoxes that may forever elude precise resolution. From this acceptance or faith may arise enhanced power for action.

HYPNOTIZABILITY

Hypnotizability can be defined loosely as ability to experience such phenomena, generally termed "hypnotic," as comfort with automaticity of behavior, vividness and freedom of imagination, and flexibility of the cognitive modalities the subject can employ. Human beings vary greatly in hypnotizability, as in the nearly infinite facets of their unique personalities. A "good" subject is generally one who is highly hypnotizable; a "poor" subject is one who is not.

Although the circularity is obvious, this does point to a dimension of human life worth careful study. This loose and quasi-circular definition refers primarily to hypnotizability as understood by hypnotherapists in clinical practice, where the therapist willingly assumes the burden of responsibility for maximizing the subject's benefits from the experience.

Since techniques are individualized and often quite imaginative, it is nearly impossible to apply the strict measurement and testing required by the scientific method. Like most medicine, clinical hypnosis is an art. Although when effective it is often difficult to know for certain exactly what it was that worked, results are sufficiently impressive to reinforce its use. To the clinician, accepting the burden of responsibility himself, the degree of hypnotizability of a subject is not as relevant as ways and means of helping him experience his assets and abilities to the fullest.

Hence, hypnotizability has received little formal study by clinicians, who more often will simply accept it as one of the many given personality traits with which to work. Erickson (Beahrs, 1971) has summarized the task of the clinical hypnotist, identical to that of the psychotherapist, in a threefold maxim:

1) Meet the patient at his own level and gain rapport. This can be rephrased as "joining the patient's system," as opposed to having him join that of the therapist. To a hypnotist this necessarily involves rapport with aspects of consciousness not usually overtly experienced—unperceived consciousness or what Erickson called "communication with the unconscious." Only by so doing can the subject feel safe responding at any other level than his customary conscious one. To feel safe, as required for the experience of automaticity and flexibility, the subject's conscious executive functions must be at ease as well. Hence the need for a hypnotherapist to have skill in dealing simultaneously with frequently discordant multiple levels of consciousness in a constructive way that is comforting on all levels.

2) Second is the need to modify the patient's productions to gain control. Control—the extent to which one can influence another or create feelings and/or behaviors different from what they otherwise would be—is a hotly argued topic in psychiatry. Most hypnotherapists accept the apparent contradiction that only the subject can really determine his own behavior, the hypnotist having no actual power to do somebody else's thing. Yet the hypnotist's capacity for influence is considerable and his responsibility for its optimal

use inescapable. It follows that, after the hypnotherapist has become part of the patient's system through gaining rapport—the first step of this process, if he subsequently changes his own behavior the patient too must change.

3) The control established during the second part of the process must be used so effectively that those changes which will necessarily occur will do so in a desirable direction. At the simple level of inducing hypnotic behavior, effective change is merely achieving comfort, safety, and facility in the hypnotic experience. Of greater relevance to the mental health professional is Erickson's claim, supported by most hypnotherapists, including myself, that the very same skills of an effective hypnotist are those of effectual psychotherapy.

A so-called "good" hypnotist is defined as a clinician with better than average skill at helping even "poor" subjects maximally experience and utilize the hypnotic dimensions of life. This involves skill in achieving rapport and communication with many levels of consciousness simultaneously. A practitioner blessed with what is known as a "therapeutic personality" can do this almost automatically. Watkins (1978) uses the term "resonance" for the process of covert multilevel rapport and communication; his volume on the subject, *The Therapeutic Self,* is an indispensable reference for those desiring detailed study in this process.

Since a research scientist is more interested in finding out what is happening than in inducing change, subject-to-subject variations in hypnotizability are more his province for study than the clinician's. To him, the burden of responsibility for achieving hypnosis rests with the subject, so that controls are established rendering subject variables measurable and testable. The chief vehicle is the standardized hypnotic susceptibility scale, of which there are many versions. Most representative are the Stanford Hypnotic Susceptibility Scales (SHSSs) of Weitzenhoffer and Hilgard (1959), many modifications of which have been made since their introduction to deal with specialized studies.

The SHSSs and related instruments are comprised of a standard hypnotic induction, read word for word, including 10 to 12 hypnotic test suggestions that cover the gamut of the three dimensions within which hypnosis is defined. As defined by these tests, hypnotizability depends upon the number of suggestions the subject responds to sufficiently for his or her response to be defined as hypnotic by a criterion level. By this measure a good subject is one who, regardless of the skill and experience of the hypnotist, will respond well to the verbatim hypnosis session. I earlier suggested (Beahrs and Humiston, 1974) that what is measured by this type of test is the subject's ability to achieve Erickson's three criteria for successful therapy—rapport, control, and change. Ability to join the therapist's system at the therapist's level indicates a type of internal malleability or adaptability most of us would consider a prime attribute of mental health.

Most clinicians discount standardized research tests, contending that any subject can experience deep levels of hypnosis if treated with sufficient skill. I have found to my satisfaction (Beahrs and Humiston, 1974) that sensory awareness approaches will facilitate deep hypnosis in some subjects scoring nearly zero on standardized inductions, though I can hardly lay claim to having achieved deep hypnosis in every instance. Modification of hypnotizability is, in fact, an area of considerable controversy among researchers. Contrary to common sense and to what the more presumptuous hypnotists would like to believe, research-style hypnotizability is a remarkably stable personality trait, perhaps more so than body weight or color of hair. Few subjects tested in the laboratory are able to increase their hypnotic responses above a certain plateau level, although there are rare exceptions where a formerly poor subject becomes a hypnotic virtuoso.

The issue in contention is whether hypnotizability is a trait or a skill. If the former, it is basically unmodifiable. The best a skilled clinician can then accomplish would be removal of whatever blocks or inhibitions prevent maximum utilization of the inherent trait within limits that cannot be exceeded. If a skill, the implication is that a subject can, as with any athletic or artistic skill, continue to improve with training, practice and patience.

Whether hypnotizability is a trait or a skill is unresolved. I personally believe that, like sports and art, it involves both. To what degree each is involved is not particularly relevant to the clinician, except to the extent that high or low hypnotizability might correlate with different types of psychiatric syndromes. On the basis of personal observation, research, and clinical experience, I do believe that people differ profoundly in intrinsic hypnotizability. Whether the cause is biological (trait), socially acquired (skill) or other, this variability, like other individual differences, must be accepted as a basic given in the therapeutic situation.

E. R. Hilgard (1968) maintains that there is little, if any, correlation between hypnotizability and psychiatric syndromes, or between hypnotizability and character types. When healthy, compulsive, hysteric, or schizophrenic groups are tested, the percentage of good, poor, and average subjects is similar. J.R. Hilgard (1970) studied the backgrounds of good subjects and found a positive correlation with permission to enjoy freedom of fantasy life.

Most pertinent to unity and multiplicity is a certain type of "difficult patient" who, when considered within the traditional psychiatric framework, challenges the resources of even the most skilled psychotherapist. Ignoring the theory but tapping my experience with hypnosis, I may perceive such a patient as functioning almost continuously in a hypnotized manner, though in so disordered a way that he is usually labeled as severely disturbed. By handling this problem as a misused hypnotic skill, it may be possible, merely by teaching the patient or giving him permission and information to use autohypnosis to his benefit, to bypass the psychopathology model entirely.

Like a knife, gun, oil or atomic energy, hypnotic ability is powerful stuff; it can be used well or poorly. Assisting the patient to use his skill well is, in principle, all that needs doing. That which was once a symptom becomes a skill.

Frankel (1976) suggested that much psychotherapy might be bypassed by the patient's learning to take charge of spontaneous hypnotic behavior when it has appeared as a symptom. This can be assisted by the therapist's using hypnotic techniques. I believe that this process applies not only to specific symptoms, but also to major psychiatric syndromes. Where this has worked, all such cases have revealed themselves as virtuoso subjects, capable of the most advanced hypnotic experience with the slightest effort. If hypnotizability is a basic trait, its use as a coping mechanism for stresses would only be available to high hypnotizables or good subjects. Looking on hypnotizability as positive, as most hypnotists do, these particular patients are fortunate; they retain the potential for rapid change.

Hypnosis will shortly be seen as the essence of unity and multiplicity. It involves simultaneous multilevel co-consciousness (a type of splitting), as well as some expansive identification with the beyond, outside the usual confines of self. Hypnotizability would then refer to facility in both splitting and expanding. The immense potential inherent in such an ability has both advantages and liabilities apparent to even the psychiatrically naive. Difficult patients exemplifying these issues are then the highly hypnotizables.

Although I do not understand why some have this trait or skill more than others, I accept it as a given fact, devoting attention here to those patients who exemplify the principles of unity and multiplicity basic to this book.

HYPNOSIS AS MULTIPLICITY—HIDDEN OBSERVERS

That some aspect or part of a hypnotized person might experience things differently from the hypnotized self was hinted many years ago by Lundeholm (1928) in studies of hypnotic deafness. The preliminary hypnotic suggestion included words to the effect that deafness could occur or not depending upon a verbal cue. Since this suggestion was followed by the subject, it was assumed that something within him must have been hearing, though he was deaf; otherwise no response could have been made to the verbal cue. Considering this merely as an observation of interest, no attempt was made to ascertain what that something was.

Orne (1959) exhaustively compared the behavior of highly hypnotizable and hypnotized subjects to that of non-hypnotizable subjects instructed to behave as if they were. The simulators became so skilled that they could fool even experienced investigators into believing they were actually hypnotized. The rationale for his study was to eliminate from the essence of hypnosis anything which could even conceivably be due to experimental artifact, such as the "demand characteristics" of the experimental setting—desire of the subject to please the hypnotist. That simulators can successfully mimic real hypnosis does not disprove its validity but simply shows that we do not know whether the behavior involved is relevant to its essence. Any differences between simulators and bonafide subjects can actually provide potent evidence for what constitutes the true essence of hypnosis as opposed to possible artifact. The most consistent finding was a type of internal reality contradiction found only in real subjects, which Orne termed "trance logic," a single example of which will serve to illustrate emerging multiplicity.

Both hypnotized subjects and simulators were given the suggestion that a certain individual standing in the room was not there, a negative hallucination. When a third individual was positioned directly behind the second, the subject was asked to walk to him with the negatively hallucinated second person directly in his path. The simulator did as would be expected of one who believed he should not be seeing the second person, bumping right into him. Although the hypnotized subject really did not see that person, he respectfully and unobtrusively walked around the obstacle, while giving every appearance of not seeing what he must actually have "seen" at another level.

Who sees and who does not? Here, in a nutshell, is a phenomenon illustrating what Hilgard (1977) was later to term the "hidden observer" and Watkins and Watkins (1979a,b) ego states or "latent alter-personalities." Multiplicity is now in the forefront.

In an attempt to determine whether some part of a hypnotically anesthetized subject might still feel pain, Hilgard and Hilgard (1975) asked such a subject to allow a finger to rise if he did, indeed, feel pain. A finger rose. When they then asked to speak with that part, they found it able to describe what was actually happening, regardless of whether reality distortions of the hypnotic experience were accepted by the subject. What Hilgard (1977) now called a hidden observer was able to demonstrate pure reality-testing analogous to an objective scientist, what transactional analysts call an uncontaminated Adult. Further, this was far more marked than customary for that particular subject, even in his usual non-hypnotic waking state.

Hilgard found that the easiest way to talk to a hidden observer was simply to ask to speak to it, as one would to a particular individual in a group. That part would then "come out" and talk. It could also be accessed by a hypnotic signal or could give a retrospective account of prior experiences matching the data by using hypnotic age regression. Implications of the hidden observer are far-flung, suggesting the probability that we have not only a conscious and an unconscious, but more than one simultaneously conscious personality, each with its own independent but fully awake subjective experience, feelings and thoughts.

Early in the nineteenth century, after successfully performing major surgery on nearly a hundred patients using only hypnotic suggestion for anesthesia, Esdaile (1846) observed that many had no recollection of anything resembling surgical pain before, during or after surgery. Yet we now know from Hilgard's work that a hidden observer really did experience the pain and could have reported it if contacted after the fact, though this awareness was entirely unconscious.

As for the hidden observer, considered a person in his own right, suppose we took one of Esdaile's patients 20 years later, hypnotized him, and accessed and talked with that observer. Had he experienced the pain? Was it a conscious experience? And did he remember it? I suspect the answer to all these questions would be yes.

It seems impossible to avoid the dilemma of a consciousness that is always unconscious or an unconscious with a conscious experience of its own all the time. It sounds like major personality splitting. And, in fact, Hilgard (1977) likened the hidden observer to those secondary personalities seen in patients with severe dissociative disorder. While the hidden observer knows both his own experience and that of the hypnotized subject, the latter knows nothing of the former — a one-way amnesic barrier often seen in multiple personality.

Watkins and Watkins (1979a) explored the hidden observer phenomenon still further, using as subjects a number of psychiatrically healthy college student volunteers. Adopting Hilgard's method, they accessed the observer for a hypnotically anesthetized subject and, as in making a new friend, went one step further by asking his name and eliciting opinions on himself and the subject's overall usual self. Often the hidden observer showed unique personality features of its own, had experiences and opinions about life quite different from the usual self. Watkins then gave the subject a different hypnotic suggestion, such as a vivid hallucinatory experience. When the hidden observer was again contacted, it proved to be an altogether different entity, with different personality traits and life views and preferring a different mode of address.

Bearing in mind that these subjects were all psychiatrically healthy individuals, the implication stated explicitly by the Watkins' is that we are all covert multiple personalities. Though not understood in the pathological sense in which the term is used in psychiatry, this may shed light on that area. Conversely, a study of psychiatric multiple personalities may help elucidate the multiplicity of consciousness that now appears to be present in all healthy living—a consideration I will discuss in detail in a later chapter.

It follows that dissociation must in some ways be essential to healthy functioning. Also, what we mean by the unconscious now becomes relative, depending upon which part-self we are communicating with. To each part, only the others may appear unconscious.

Hypnosis involves unity and multiplicity at the other end of the continuum as well. Not only does a hypnotic subject manifest split-off part-selves with their own consciousness, but there is also a sense in which the subject expands, extends or merges beyond his usual self boundaries into his environment. Freud (1920), an experienced and sophisticated hypnotist, hypothesized that hypnosis is similar to love. In both, the subject loosens his ego boundaries and extends his sense of selfhood to include another—in hypnosis, the hypnotist; in love, the love object. In both cases the subject's sense of selfhood and power for action are paradoxically increased by this merging, contrary to the symbiotic psychoses where a similar process leads to a drastic reduction in reality-testing and coping.

To Freud, inclusion of the hypnotist in a subject's self boundaries adequately explained the subject's acceptance of hypnotic suggestion as his own. It does not, however, make clear why the resultant action is experienced as automatic rather than as a voluntary free choice. Hilgard's neodissociation model explains better why a hand levitation, for example, carries the illusion of just happening. If the part-self voluntarily lifting the hand is different from the one in primary conscious control, the conscious self will experience the other part as unconscious and its actions as involuntary or spontaneous. Hypnosis seems to illustrate dissociation or differentiation in conjunction with expansion or extension. If only one part of the subject's psyche is in rapport with the hypnotist and following his suggestions, another part has an illusion of automaticity. Giving the hypnotic suggestion to a hidden part of the subject illustrates Erickson's "communication with the unconscious."

Gill and Brenman (1959) expanded on Freud's psychoanalytic model, arriving at a concept of hypnosis as a "regression in the service of the ego." The capacity for full use of primitive cognitive modes (regression) has been included in our three-factor definition of hypnosis; its enhancement of mental strength (in the service of the ego) cannot be overemphasized. Basing their theory on clinical observation, the authors note that during transition into hypnosis a subject may momentarily experience "transition phenomena," including intense affect and even abreaction, laughing or crying, and a transitory loosening in ability to think clearly. When the hypnotic state is established, the transitory disorganization resolves and the ego becomes reorganized into new subsystems in rapport with the hypnotist. These are split off from the part of the subject's usual reality ego, which correctly experiences the hypnotic behavior as occurring outside its own control.

Splitting and extending of the subject's ego boundaries occur simultaneously within hypnosis. This is also compatible with what is found in the psychoanalytic models, and correlates well enough with recent research data that I find no need to pit the latter against the former. This is a particularly interesting interpretation in the light of certain conclusions within the psychoanalytic discipline, based on study of those patients for whom exactly these two processes—splitting and symbiotic extension of ego boundaries—define their very pathology. These are the narcissistic and borderline personalities being reformulated by psychoanalysts like Kernberg (1975) and Kohut (1971).

Yet, these are precisely the same psychiatric entities I have likened to spontaneous hypnosis in the hope of encouraging a treatment paradigm in which what was once a symptom can become a skill. Here may be a bridge between hypnosis, psychoanalysis and the issues of unity and multiplicity in all life.

It seems to me that hypnosis research, increasingly redundant, keeps returning to a few core issues we are so far from understanding that for now we must accept them as givens. One is the ability to imagine so vividly that we may even perceive our imaginings, what Sheehan and Perry (1976) see as the prime factor into which all hypnosis research is dovetailing. Another is the "regressive" component or Frankel's (1976) "trance as a coping mechanism," suggesting that when faced with a problem we might simply tap the nearly infinite resources within the inner self for help. This issue is the only one which may find an explanation within psychodynamic models.

More relevant to this inquiry are such issues as divisions of consciousness, extension into the beyond, voluntary versus involuntary action, and the nature of executive function in life, all of which I will address in considerable detail after presenting two cases illustrating spontaneous hypnosis.

3

Spontaneous Hypnotic Behavior as Symptom or Skill

Two actual cases effectively illustrate automatic hypnotic behavior as it can occur in everyday life. The first shows it as a potent and life-saving coping mechanism. The second shows how this function, when gone awry, may lead to severe disturbance challenging the resources of most psychiatrists. Seeing it simply as misused ability, appropriate therapeutic intervention involves taking charge of the disorder so it can become, as in the first case, the useful coping mechanism it should be.

CASE 1. SPONTANEOUS TRANCE BEHAVIOR IN MENTAL HEALTH

Mr. X, an experienced 24-year-old mountaineer, found himself in an untenable situation during a mountain climb, partly through overexuberance and partly by simple misfortune. He was alone, though by prearrangement barely an hour ahead of a large, organized climbing party. He was slightly off route. To his left was a 1000-foot drop-off onto a crevassed glacier; to his right and above, a high-angled slope of rock sufficiently loose and "cruddy" that further uphill climbing would be at his peril.

39

The misfortune was a sudden rockslide from his approach route, rendering strategic withdrawal an untenable option. The perch itself being somewhat precarious, our protagonist now faced imminent danger of sudden death. He subsequently reported sequential changes in his state of mind sufficiently striking to warrant discussion.

As his retreat route was closed off by the rockslide, he immediately perceived his peril with full cognitive awareness, though his first reaction was hardly predicted upon rational inquiry. "You stupid #$%8ᶜ!!!, you've done it again!! When in the !⁹#$% are you ever going to start using that brain God put into that thick skull of yours?!!!" Not only the Critical Parent of transactional analysis, but pure rage.

Only moments later it was, "Well, I guess this is it. We all have to go sooner or later, and it looks as if my time has come. I have a lot more I'd like to experience in life, but what I've done already has made it worthwhile." Along with these thoughts came a profound, almost ineffable sense of peaceful relaxation of body and mind, during which Mr. X reviewed many long "forgotten" early experiences. While no more than two or three minutes passed by actual clock time, his experience was one of many hours of elapsed time, a major time expansion.

Then, again as if it just happened, another ego state shift occurred, this time into a clear-headed, emotionally impassive, objective scientist type, the pure Adult of T.A. "Well, I'm not dead yet, and won't be for a while as long as I stay put. So let's look at my options, at all possibilities, and assess the benefit/detriment factors of each." He decided to stay put as long as he could and await rescue by the approaching climbing party from below. He decided on the least risky escape plan he would institute if he first became too dangerously tired. Forty-five minutes of clock time elapsed before he was indeed rescued, although it seemed that he waited only two or three minutes, a major time contraction. He gratefully completed the ascent with his companions.

To a psychiatrist experienced with unusual coping mechanisms, hypnosis and altered states of consciousness, several features of the process described stand out. First, the fear—probably abject terror—that must have been there at some level was never consciously experienced until after his rescue when it was literally safe to be afraid. There were a few deep breaths, a "Thank God, it's great to be alive" feeling, and then onward. The following week he slept only fitfully, however, being interrupted by frequent nightmares of meeting a violent ending, not only by accident but also by several other means he had scared himself with at various points in his life. This mild post-traumatic neurosis subsided after about a week, as life continued with a more mature sense of its meaning and value.

Thinking hypnotically, the unconscious (or one of its component parts) must have sensed immediately the danger of a fear or panic reaction and chose to handle the situation on its own. It first dissociated the fear out of awareness where it could do no harm, then later worked it through by an extensive process of dreaming. Since the conscious self was not deprived of any of the fruits of awareness, he could in a sense enjoy the best of both worlds. Dynamically, this is an example in a normal healthy person of what resembles a secondary alter-personality taking over when conditions warrant it.

Thinking in terms of normal dissociation and the syntax of his internal dialogue, how this individual addressed himself is of interest. In the first, angry ego state it was in second person — "You stupid idiot!" — as if talking to another person. In both the second stage (peace of mind, acceptance of death as well as life) and the third (objective assessment), he used the first person "I" with full experience of self-hood. The first response was like a secondary personality coming out — one clearly different from the internal self helper or unconscious who presumably was the executor of the entire operation. Transactional analysts note frequent use of the second person when coming from a "Parent" ego state, an observation worth further exploration.

Since time distortion is a common feature of hypnotic experience, observing this is one of the best indices of when spontaneous hypnosis is occurring, whether in the therapist-client relationship or everyday life. Both expansion and contraction of time were experienced in this instance, each in such a way as to enhance likelihood of survival, maximize the possible experiential learning and keep pain and suffering to a bare minimum. All are adaptive. Frankel (1976) refers to trance as a coping mechanism, and I can hardly think of a better illustration.

The stage of relaxed resignation had profound experiential learning significance though relatively little immediate protective value. Hence it was expanded in subjective time so that one minute seemed an hour or more. The ensuing period of prolonged waiting, potentially exhausting but calling for no further creative thinking, was conversely contracted in subjective time, perceived as the briefest of interludes.

Considered for its adaptive value, the sequential progression of ego states and moods is also of interest. The first response may have been of value more in the mood than in the self-critical context, though critical self-assessment was certainly indicated after the fact. Early researchers describe the organism's response to survival threat as either fight or flight, both reactions mediated by the sympathetic nervous system. In the above circumstances, flight, triggered by a fear or panic reaction, would have meant immediate death. While less predictable, the rage response mobilized that aggressive and desperately needed problem-solving energy that enables men and women to rise to acts of heroism beyond their usual selves in crises such as war and natural disaster.

Once energy was mobilized, it was necessary to relax, leading to that state of effortless hypervigilance which is at the core of great athletic performance. Time expansion enabled Mr. X to rapidly survey nearly his entire life history, though expending little precious clock time. This relaxed phase somewhat resembles hypnotic trance, though we know by now that the domain of hypnosis goes far beyond this caricature. A colleague has also likened it to the "death experience," as described by many diverse sources. In any case, ability to foster a more relaxed aggressive position and receptivity to objective information-processing was ultimately the decisive factor in this individual's having survived and profited by his experience.

Hilgard emphasizes that the dissociative split occurring in healthy hypnotic subjects seems structurally the same as what is observed in multiple personalities. In his terminology, that part of Mr. X which took over and assumed executive control of the operation without his conscious awareness of it would be called a hidden observer. Allison (1974) would call it an internal self helper. Watkins and Watkins (1979a) suggested that hidden observers are actually latent alter-personalities with their own defining characteristics that collectively make up an individual's "personality"; they maintain that we are all at least latent multiple personalities.

That the subject of this narrative was in a spontaneous hypnotic trance by virtually all our stated criteria is hard to dispute. That it was adaptive is evidenced by both his survival and the absence of more "normal" responses such as fear that could have spelled disaster. I fully believe that most surviving individuals could supply example upon example of situations in which their unconscious took over with much better results than could have accrued from conscious trying. Even the majority of consciously self-destructive suicidal patients will save themselves, usually without awareness of how, as would appear from the 10:1 ratio of reported attempts to actual suicides. I doubt that it would be all that difficult to die if one wanted to *at all levels.*

Transient amnesic episodes occasionally accompany hypnotic problem-solving, and this may frighten a subject into a psychiatrist's office. Yet, the point I want to emphasize is that hypnosis is an adaptive skill, an ability (Hilgard, 1968). Capacity for even spontaneous hypnosis is not only adaptive but can be life-saving, as the above vignette and countless others illustrate. Cultivation of unconscious problem-solving ability is hardly to be discounted. I find the clearest description of this process in lay terms in Gallwey's book, *Inner Tennis* (1976).

What we psychiatrists have still hardly touched upon is why not *all* individuals go into spontaneous trance that is truly in the service of the ego or overall self. The multiplicity model as posed by the episode on the mountain may explain a great deal, though by no means all. Why does one individual, like the above, automatically give executive control to his most competent part when desperately needed, while another person may not? Another young adventurer, of comparable or greater mental health, in a similar crisis might access a terrified child, with death the tragic result. Even sadder is knowing that he, like Mr. X, had somewhere within his unconscious what he needed to save himself. Why he gave executive control to the wrong ego state I do not know. While "covert suicide" is probably a factor in many accidental deaths, this was apparently not the case here. Can preventive parenting and/or preventive psychiatry, in a way not yet clear, do something to help one develop the best crisis-solving priorities so they just happen instantly when needed?

CASE 2. A SKILL AS A SYMPTOM AND AGAIN A SKILL

Some years ago I was called to attend Mrs. R, who appeared in a hospital emergency room acutely psychotic. She did not appear to see or hear anyone present, was disoriented to time and place, whimpering and crying like a small child in distress and talking with somebody or something that was not seen or heard by any other personnel actually present. Though only in her mid-thirties, she had carried the stigma of a long-term diagnosis of schizophrenia, with many acute episodes apparently similar to the one at hand. Massive doses of Thorazine (approximately 1,200 mg. per day) had been used for both sedating and antipsychotic effects without any significant response. She had also suffered a range of bizzare and severe medical symptoms that had eluded diagnostic evaluation, so she was not only "schizo" but also a schizophrenic "crock" — and visibly suffering to boot.

My immediate reaction, tapping prior experience not only with "real" schizophrenics but also, fortunately, with normal hypnosis, was essentially that this woman was not schizophrenic. She did not show any of Bleuler's (1911) four As — loosening of associations, autism, flattening of affect, and social or emotional ambivalence — acting rather more like a desperate tiny child. She appeared to be seeing, hearing and talking to someone not only perceived at the time (hallucination) but also apparently actually perceived at some critical time in her childhood.

Was this a case of spontaneous hypnotic age regression that fit all Mrs. R's current symptoms? At the moment the reason was irrelevant. My chief priority was to find out what to do about it. Since she could not see or hear us, Mrs. R was apparently wholly out of contact. But was she? Or was there some part or aspect of her, I wondered, that even while regressed could hear me and respond? At least I could try to make contact. (Had I at that point been fully aware of the definitive works of Hilgard and Watkins, an affirmative answer to my question would have been obvious.)

I recalled Erickson's threefold maxim for effective indirect hypnotic interventions (Beahrs 1971): Gain rapport with the patient at (in this case) her present level, becoming part of her system; modify her productions, gaining control; and use that control in such a way that the change necessarily occurring will be in a desirable direction. Simply talking with Mrs. R as if I had actually been a hypnotist who suggested her original regression, I conducted myself like a hypnotist in rapport with a regressed subject, giving hypnotic suggestions of my own to which she responded.

Within 20 minutes the situation was phenomenologically indistinguishable from any experimental age regression with a good hypnotic subject. The patient accepted the suggestion that her hypnotic skill was indeed a skill that she could use when needed under her full voluntary control. Except for a fleeting one-minute episode shortly thereafter, the psychosis never recurred. What was once a symptom had indeed become a skill — and in a space of barely 20 minutes.

This patient was hardly cured in a characterological sense. She was now best described as a highly immature and/or hysterical personality who had great difficulty in relating with other adults in a truly adult-to-adult manner. Her psychotic episodes were indeed psychotic and she had been out of touch with current reality in an exceedingly disabling manner. But she had never been schizophrenic.

Her condition was more like spontaneous hypnosis not in the service of the ego, though more literally serving it in an unsatisfactory way. Her adult coping skills were so limited that the spontaneous regressions could be seen as her unconscious taking over when knowing that her usual self could not cut the mustard. Probably quite similar in mechanism to the experience of the mountaineer, this is, however, less adaptive. While the personality disorder required more than three years of ego-building psychotherapy, Mrs. R was actually cured of the originally alarming psychotic episodes in that initial 20 minutes. This remarkable woman became one of the most skilled virtuoso hypnotic subjects I have ever worked with.

Of additional interest was her ability to report accurately in a subsequent hypnotic regression some rather grisly talk heard while she was anesthetized during surgery, at which time the surgeons had discovered considerable evidence that many of her earlier medical symptoms were not entirely "in her head," despite her being at the top of the class in imaginative abilities in a basically hysterical character. Most experienced hypnotherapists can recount similar case histories touching upon the operating room. Physicians of all specialties should realize that many — and possibly most — anesthetized patients do process information concerning what is going on during an operation at a time when they are particularly vulnerable to misinterpreting verbal transactions.

In my last contact with her, I found Mrs. R doing well. But ever since that initial 20 minutes, I personally have not been the same. Although I have yet to work with another person so classic for spontaneous trance, by keeping my third eye and ear open I have found num-

erous instances in which spontaneous hypnotic behavior that is not
adaptive has been misdiagnosed as major mental illness, with resultant years of tragic, unnecessary suffering and ineffectual treatment.
Many cases have been multiple personalities or individuals afflicted
with severe ego state disorders; however, it seems that spontaneous
trance can cover almost as wide a range of psychiatric symptomatology as psychiatry itself. Obsessive-compulsive syptoms certainly bear
a resemblance to a subject's carrying out a post-hypnotic suggestion,
for example. A depressive neurosis may be the presentation of only
the primary personality in a dissociation syndrome, with the larger
portion of the patient's personality being hidden beyond awareness
with a dissociative barrier.

The only two ways I know for a psychiatrist to become accurate in
these diagnoses are: 1) by gaining sufficient experience with hypnosis
to recognize it in this spontaneously occurring form that is doing such
disservice to the ego; and 2) by becoming more precise in the defining
criteria of other major mental disorders, such as schizophrenia and
manic-depressive states. It would also be wise to take another close
look at patients who do not respond to traditional treatment.

DYSFUNCTIONAL HYPNOTIC BEHAVIOR

On the face of it, disorders resembling hypnotic behavior not in the
service of the ego appear as a symptom instead of the skill that they
can and should be — and, in a sense, always are. These fall naturally
into three categories in the areas of volition, perception and recall.

Disorders of Volition

Paralleling hypnotic motor phenomena, disorders of volition include hysterical paralyses and some spontaneous immobilizations like
catatonia, on the one hand — often phenomenologically identical to
simple hypnotic test responses — and such movement disorders as hysterical seizures, on the other hand. More than one such patient has
learned to "throw a fit" intentionally so that a symptom has become a
skill.

At a higher level, any complex behavior pattern which is experienced as involuntary, "not-me" or "it" could be considered similar in

kind. Haley (1963) has defined a psychiatric symptom as a "power tactic," used by a patient as an unusual strategy to cope with a problem that had appeared insurmountable. Within the limits of relevance of this concept, my idea of taking charge of a symptom so it becomes a skill merges inextricably with the strategic therapies of Haley and the brief therapy mode of the Palo Alto group (Watzlawick, Weakland, and Fisch, 1974).

Disorders of Perception

These include both time distortion and such somatic misperception as hysterical anesthesias, paresthesias and hyperesthesias. The experience of the mountaineer in crisis illustrated this. Whenever borderline personalities make some out-of-character remark such as "everything seems in high gear" or "in slow motion," incongruent with their outward behavior, I am at once alert for signs of a spontaneous hypnotic experience that can be taken charge of and rendered a skill. Such remarks are almost as common in borderline patients as they are in normal hypnotized subjects, suggesting even further that the processes have much in common.

Disorders of Recall

Psychogenic amnesia, fugue states and depersonalization represent a third category of dysfunctional spontaneous hypnotic behavior, though they are also capable of conversion into a therapeutic skill. These dissociative phenomena mimic behaviors that can be quite normal within a hypnotic state. They will be discussed in more detail in Chapter 5.

Most, if not all, individuals with spontaneous hypnotic behavior as a major presenting symptom fit easily into the rubric of narcissistic and borderline personality disorders, as stated by Gruenewald (1977) with regard to multiple personalities. Many therapists claim that formal psychoanalysis is the preferable if not the only treatment for these severe disorders. Yet the case of Mrs. R points out the tragedy of not at least trying a simpler way first.

The value of my current emphasis upon treating such symptoms as hypnotic, taking charge and rendering them a skill is not so much theoretical as pragmatic. Indeed, I make no pretense of matching the precision and detail of such recent psychoanalytic formulations as those of Kernberg (1975) and Kohut (1971). The merit of the approach lies in the results, for certain patients do respond dramatically to this form of treatment. And when it works, it is often remarkably fast.

HYPNOSIS AND FREUD

Just as most of today's investigators agree that hypnotic phenomena are on a continuum with non-hypnotic or everyday life, so Freud described a parallel continuum as the "Psychopathology of Everyday Life." Oddly enough, the psychiatric symptoms I compare to spontaneous hypnosis are exactly those known to have been the object of initial scrutiny by Freud — hysterical disorders that many current investigators believe were actually more narcissistic. I suspect that Freud himself must have observed the parallel I am convinced exists between these psychiatric disorders and hypnotic phenomena, for, as Kline (1972) reminds us, he was one of the most skilled hypnotherapists of his time and wrote, early in his career (1891), papers on hypnotic techniques definitive even today.

Although many reasons have been advanced for Freud's abandoning hypnosis in favor of the psychanalytic method, one plausible possibility has received scant attention. Since even today we fully comprehend neither hysterical disorders nor hypnosis, we lack a framework for that precise type of definition demanded by Freud. Not being one for pseudo-explanations, he would hardly be willing to settle for a definition in which phenomenon A is "explained" by saying it is the same as phenomenon B, about which equally little is understood. For Freud, as for his peers, complete understanding was a precondition for any power for action.

So, to the detriment of practical aspects of psychotherapy but resulting in inestimable gain to psychoanalytical understanding, Freud chose to abandon the less precise science of hypnosis to concentrate on his own breakthrough in psychoanalysis. It would be up to Milton H. Erickson, now becoming in the area of pragmatic therapeutic techniques the giant Freud is in psychoanalytic theory, to later lead the resurgence in hypnotic and strategic therapies. Freely admitting that he did not fully understand all he was able to accomplish, Erickson dismissed the importance of complete understanding. Assiduously avoiding propounding any clear theoretical system of his own for fear that it would be too limiting, he continued to practice what he insisted was simple commonsense psychology.

If A is the same as B and we know what to do with B, though we are unclear as to its precise nature, it follows, as I see it, that we must also know what to do with A. And since the work of Bernheim (1890), there has been remarkable overall consensus regarding what to do with hypnotic phenomena, despite lack of adequate theoretical understanding. Following the above logic, it follows that we should apply the time-worn proven hypnotic techniques to psychiatric disorders which are phenomenologically identical. Initial clinical results are sufficiently encouraging to suggest that this approach be explored in considerably more depth and that its limits of relevance and applicability be defined.

The value of the spontaneous trance model, then, is more practical than theoretical. Perhaps the theoretical contribution is at another level. The above provides evidence — empirical evidence — that what helps us enhance our understanding does not always correlate with what works, accomplishes desired change or enhances power for action. This suggests that the criteria for judging beliefs and belief systems may not be so much whether or not they are true, but rather, whether they work. Are they *useful?* And if so, what are their limits of relevance? In my opinion, it is especially the latter question which needs more careful defining by collective clinical experience.

4

The Executive Role in Divisions of Consciousness

I find it meaningful to define as a mental or physical *entity* only those collections of existing matter-energy with definite distinguishing boundaries from what is beyond, as well as unique intrinsic qualities and existence over a finite time span. Bearing this in mind, a *mental unit* can be defined as any consciously experiencing entity, whether a cell, part-self or human being — or even a larger aggregate mental unit as postulated by certain psychics but so far beyond scientific testing. Ultimately, the existence of any entity can be called into question when its limits of relevance are pushed (see Appendix I). Hence it is crucial to keep within these limits, especially when working with a given personality or mental unit that is hard to measure or test. This is equally so with the limits of any theoretical belief system.

That consciousness in at least some rudimentary form permeates existing reality at all levels is increasingly accepted by as diverse professionals as physicists and psychiatrists. Even so, we are as far as ever from being able to define exactly what we mean by it. By simply carrying premises acceptable to most scientists to their logical conclusion, I reached the conclusion in *That Which Is* (1977a) that energy, constituting all that exists, is *spiritual* in its primary essence. Some type of primordial consciousness is inherent, then, in any entity or organization of energy, as it experiences its own being. What then distinguishes a human mind from that of "non-sentient" organisms or entities which are still composed of the same energy, whose essence is spiritual? I used as my starting point two observations — that the basic energy of existence appears to be organized in a virtually limitless number of patterns or entities and that these fall into different orders of complexity or levels of organization.

Keenly aware that in actual fact the energy of "All That Is" blurs into one infinite continuum and that any finite entity has only indefinite and to an extent arbitrary bounds, I nonetheless attempted to show that human consciousness as we experience it depends upon perceiving and defining entities, while perforce falling far short of even approximating the whole truth. When their limits of relevance are approached, all entities become subject to the ravages of what I have been calling the A/Not-A Absurdity, opening to question even the existence of said entity. This applies not only to God, hypnosis, and multiple personalities, but even to entities whose boundaries and defining characteristics are as seemingly clear as those of a given chair or a human individual's selfhood, the boundaries of which are increasingly open to dispute within the mental health professions.

In exploring what constitutes higher thought, as opposed to the primordial spirituality of energy itself (Beahrs, 1977a), I was led to the premise that an organism capable of higher thought must be organized in such a manner as to perceive both self and external entities and to form imagery paralleling these perceptions. Essential too is a memory mechanism giving the organism a sense of continuing identity over time, though illusory in the scientific sense.

Hilgard (1977) also suggests that a strong memory mechanism is a primary prerequisite for what we call consciousness. Cohesive self is even defined psychoanalytically (Kohut, 1971) as that which experiences itself as a mental and physical unit with extension in space and continuity in time. The word *experience* should be underscored to emphasize that the unique identity does not imply any absolute wholeness or suggest estrangement from either its own parts or from All That Is. While selfhood constitutes unique humanness, it is ultimately no more absolute than the concept of hypnotic trance. Both are invaluable and both lead to absurdity when attempting total precision in separating what is "A" from what is not.

I do not know of any psychological or neurophysiological data or theory which explains or even defines consciousness. My tentative working model (Beahrs 1977a) remains as satisfactory as any to me for philosophical purposes, if it is simply modified to include a mechanism for multilevel co-consciousness within the same brain. Yet, even with this, I am unable to give any but a primary definition of consciousness as a basic given like "exist" or "spiritual."

To say a pattern of energy in our brains is conscious only if neurologically active would ignore data from both hypnosis and psychoanalysis illustrating the power and activity of unconscious cognitions. To consider consciousness only as that over which we have free choice runs counter to awareness of obsessive intrusions, ideas or automatic impulses we might prefer to rid ourselves of. Even temporal continuity, a continual memory mechanism, runs into trouble in study of amnesic states, for a sense of temporal continuity persists even when there are breaks in the flow of awareness, as in sleep. And in situations where we experience temporal breaks, like chemical and hypnotic amnesias, memory can often be recalled after the fact via hypnotic regression. To define consciousness as awareness does little more than define *exist* as *to be* (Beahrs, 1977a); though a tautology, it does point beyond itself to a dimension of experience that cannot be defined in other measurable terms, but must be accepted as a given — what I had referred to as a primary definition.

It appears that all mental activity is really conscious and that when we talk of the (or an) unconscious we must be referring to something conscious at another level. It is generally agreed that an individual can consciously experience himself but not another; the mental experience of the other can only be inferred from his behavior. In other words, another person's experience is unconscious for oneself. If different personalities experientially discrete from one another exist within a single individual, what is consciously experienced by one might be unconscious for another. While this may appear quasi-mystical to the scientifically-minded reader, I should note that simultaneous co-consciousness is the only way I know to avoid the logical absurdity (A/Not-A) into which scientific precision would otherwise unavoidably lead us — a conclusion already seen to have support from certain hard data provided by hypnotic research (see Appendix I).

In discussing mental states further, I will be implicitly following a basic working model abstracted from as diverse sources as developmental cognitive psychology (Piaget) (Flavell, 1963), psychoanalysis (Freud), and neurophysiology (Hebb). Keeping this as simple as possible, I see our minds as a composite of mental units or schemata organized in hierarchical levels of organization of complexity. To some degree it is useful to distinguish thoughts or cognitions resembling mental structures or entities from affects or drives that are more like mental forces or psychic energy. Hebb's (1949) concept of drive force as cognitive disorganization is still appealing to me and even harkens back to Spinoza's (1677) definition of emotion as a "confused idea," though I doubt that this is the only way to look upon the data adequately. If we assume only one or two basic forms of drive tension, libido and aggression for example, then more complex derivative drives are combinations and displacements of these onto increasingly complex cognitive structures. As in natural evolution, higher types of thought and behavior patterns (or mental units) develop only after the next lower. In other words, mental development must occur in stages of graded complexity — what I have called the "stage rule" and which in psychiatry is called "epigenesis."

Turning now to a discussion of psychoanalytic models of consciousness and the unconscious and recent conceptions of vertical and horizontal splits of consciousness, I will show how these dovetail with results of hypnosis research to suggest the inevitability of multiple consciousness, inherent in individual "unity."

HORIZONTAL SPLITTING—THE FREUDIAN UNCONSCIOUS AND REPRESSION BARRIERS

Psychoanalytic theory of development and mental function, as originally formulated by Freud (1916), can, in its most common interpretation, be schematized as in Figure 1. Mental development is perceived as a pyramid with the apex down. Humans begin life, as infants or even earlier, with one or possibly two types of barely differentiated drive tension and a few built-in schemata or mental units for actions, such as crying, sucking and sleeping. In the absence of signifi-

cant cognitive structures or organizations, infants are utterly at the
mercy of outside forces to satisfy their needs and provide what cannot
be provided by their own efforts. Such forces are termed "parental"
and contain nourishing and behavior-limiting aspects, both of which
are necessary for sustaining life.

As a child develops, the elaboration of progressively more complex
mental abilities allows a correspondingly more elaborate ability to
solve his own problems. On the diagram, each circle represents a
mental unit, those at a more complex level schematized by a collection of circles (as within the dotted oval) which might comprise multiple thoughts and coping mechanisms over even more than one stage

Figure 1
The Psychoanalytic Model—1

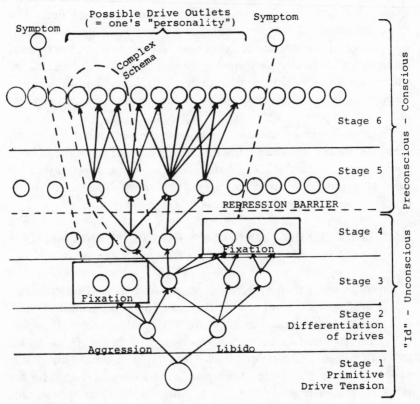

of cognitive development. Ideally, through mechanisms such as displacement and sublimation, an individual continues to develop mental units that can be employed to face whatever situation the vicissitudes of life subject him to.

At each higher stage of development, new coping mechanisms appear, allowing more autonomy by supplying a greater number of alternatives applicable to any given problem situation. The multiplicity of mental units at the top of the diagram illustrates the greater freedom and flexibility available as one learns and develops, with more options for handling any one life problem. With more choice, it is far more likely that a well-developed or "healthy" individual will be able to solve even difficult, stressful issues and continue to grow. There is, besides, less likelihood that he will run out of mature solutions and have to regress to outgrown or outmoded coping mechanisms appropriate only at an early age. Both advantages reflect what psychiatrists term "ego strength."

Nobody quite achieves this ideal. When a crisis in development is accompanied by so much stress as to surpass the organism's limits of tolerance, the individual may simply avoid the problem area by escaping to more conflict-free areas, isolating or walling off the area of stress from the mainstream of his or her mental life. Often a conscious choice at first, sooner or later this response escapes voluntary control. Now "fixated" and incapable of further development, the conflicted area cannot be activated to consciousness no matter how hard the individual may try (though it gains conscious experience within the dream state and can be activated by hypnosis and intensive psychoanalysis).

The resultant developmental arrest or fixation can be maintained by at least two mechanisms. First, since the conflict was accompanied by such overwhelming anxiety that it was consistently avoided in the first place, any attempt to reactivate it would be opposed by the full force of the pleasure principle or drive reduction—"repression." Second, with habitual disuse, these conflicted mental units become so isolated from the mainstream of a person's actual life that there are fewer and fewer associational connections with them. This mechanism may also contribute to repression, though it is possibly even more relevant to what I will later discuss as vertical splits or dissociative barriers.

Following Freud for the moment, we assume that the walled off or fixated areas do not undergo significant further development and that their activition will be opposed by considerable mental force. They are now relegated to the unconscious, defined by Freud as that area of mental life that cannot be brought to conscious awareness by voluntary choice. The unconscious in this sense is usually a collection of primitive drives maintained "beneath" a repression barrier.

The term "horizontal" is used to denote this type of split in consciousness by virtue of its implication that what is conscious at a later or higher stage of development is above that which is not. Because of its seemingly unresolvable internal conflicts, what is repressed would necessarily include those types of mental units most threatening to us, including incestuous (oedipal) drive, unbridled homicidal aggression and the whole gamut of thoughts rejected as part of one's basic nature.

These mental units are collectively termed the id, considered a caldron of untamed primitive fury which, if given control, would threaten the integrity of the individual's peace of mind and would be destructive of his overall mental function and dangerous to society, hence to himself. The unconscious is not equated entirely with id, however. As can be seen in Figure 1, it also includes primitive structures not wholly conflicted but simply outgrown. With newer coping mechanisms becoming more effective, older ones are so seldom brought into play that they are presumably forgotten. By both aspects of this conception, the unconscious is that which is below a horizontal repression barrier.

The greater the incidence of development arrest by this model, the more an adult individual's mental health is impaired—first by having fewer mental units or options at the highest level applicable to a real life problem, hence fewer alternative behaviors and less freedom; and second, by increasing the likelihood that a mental unit useful only at an earlier stage will be reactivated. A classic example of such regression under stress is a five-year-old child who acts like a three-year-old on his first day at school.

An adult with many areas of developmental arrest lacks freedom and ego strength and is prone to regression. He is especially vulnerable in precisely those areas of life that are outgrowths of whatever was repressed. When stressed in that direction, he will regress to and attempt to activate those fixated areas, which will then be opposed by the very same defensive functions instigating them in the first place, frequently resulting in a neurotic symptom.

Experienced as ego-alien or not-me, the symptom is a compromise formation between the repressed drive and that doing the repressing. Both are expressed, though only partially and in a distorted and symbolic way incomprehensible to the individual's conscious self. While Freud clearly showed the relevance of this type of process even in normal everyday life, the consequences can be disastrous.

The task of psychoanalytic treatment is to remove the developmental arrest so that the full potential of the individual can grow and flower. Freud summarized the goal as "where Id was shall Ego be," ego referring to the collective of coping mechanisms or problem-solving abilities, including that of organizing the experience of selfhood. The task is not easy. To activate fixated areas is difficult for the very reasons they were fixated in the first place.

When the treating psychoanalyst assumes the position of a benign and competent authority, this will in itself associate with the patient's multiple attitudes and behaviors toward early parent figures. And if the analyst holds his own unique personality relatively away from view, like a blank screen, the patient will unavoidably behave and feel toward him as he did toward parent figures in early life, seeing the analyst not as he really is, but as a projection of aspects of his own formerly hidden past. In what is called *transference,* what was past and hidden is now present and active in the context of the patient's distorted relationship with his analyst. "Working through" the transference, a prime feature of the psychoanalytic method, then requires working through the conflicted areas — an indirect way of reliving and solving the early fixated life dilemmas. Some variant of this process — working through loaded and conflicted areas of a patient's mental life within the safety of a competent and ethical professional setting — underlies almost all modes of long-term therapy.

The limits of relevance of this model are still hotly debated. At one level, the processes described and illustrated in Figure 1 seem so clear as to be obvious, the one major trouble spot being our old bugaboo, the A/Not-A absurdity. Is the unconscious really unconscious? Or do all mental units that have developed during an entire life span, even those which are repressed, have some continuing conscious activity? If so, repressed features might sometimes consolidate and organize themselves into more complex and higher mental units simultaneously with that which is not repressed, to resemble a separate personality. Having a conscious experience of their own, though unconscious to the usual self, do they, in fact — contrary to a literal interpretation of the terms fixation or developmental arrest — develop to higher levels separately from the patient's usual conscious self?

If this is the case, we would then have a vertical split between two or more sectors of the personality, each comprising a hierarchy of developmental levels. The split is no longer between above and below; it is, rather, "beside." Not only does hypnosis research suggest this strongly, but such a mechanism is also proposed by Kohut (1971) to describe the type of individual experiencing problems in his sense of unity and multiplicity.

The original psychoanalytic model can be diagrammed in a second way, complementary to the first, as depicted in Figure 2. It is hoped that this will give a more balanced view of the unconscious, while staying within Freud's original framework. In contrast to Figure 1, development and mental function are here depicted as a pyramid with the apex up. The unconscious contains all memories and thoughts, experiences and coping mechanisms, including primitive ones at all levels that have long since been outgrown.

Every circle or mental unit is still present, at least in the sense that it can be reactivated by various means from hypnotic age regression to transference. Though "forgotten" by disuse atrophy, factors that are outgrown and/or rarely used remain in the unconscious, with a narrowing of conscious awareness to the most relevant life issues at hand. The more mental units or schemata one develops, the more essential is selectivity concerning which to employ. The question is whether only one train of thought can be conscious at a given time, or two or three; my personal inclination is for the greater number.

Still, consciousness can entertain but a few ideas at once, while the unconscious simultaneously handles a great and possibly infinite number. The top of the pyramid in Figure 2 illustrates what is actually conscious, in contrast to the multiple units at the top of Figure 1 illustrating what is available to consciousness by voluntary choice. Freud's reference to this as "preconscious" is included in most interpretations of the conscious mind. In any case, perceiving the uncon-

Figure 2
The Psychoanalytic Model-2
Channeling of Multiple Primitive Drives
into Directed Adult Outlets
(Sexual Development Used as Example, per Freud)

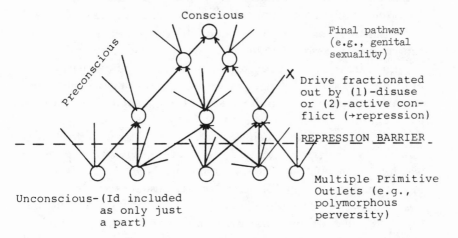

Despite multiplicity of derivative drives,   result can also
be a narrowing of acceptable outlets - yet the Unconscious
contains all the prior learnings and coping mechanisms, at
all levels.

scious as repository of all prior learning, experiences, behaviors, and coping mechanisms — along with its ability for simultaneous information-processing at potentially infinite instead of selectively limited levels — permits a conception of it, even within the Freudian framework, as a most powerful and essential force for life and growth. This concept, in contrast to the more negative id concept, is the way the unconscious is interpreted and used by hypnotherapists.

The major unresolved issue emerging from this alternative complementary picture of Freud's model is the nature of what is at the top of the pyramid. Instead of asking the nature of the unconscious, we must now ask the nature of the conscious! If we accept hypnotic data on co-consciousness and its merging with updated psychoanalytic theory, we must ask why and how this one tiny sector of a person's mental life, all of it consciously experienced at some level, seems to take primacy with respect to the individual's "usual self" and the way he is perceived by most other people. This is the problem of the *executive*, charged with determining who or what is in control of a person's behavior. Only that part of a person in executive control is able to move the voluntary skeletal muscles to implement his choices and decisions.

If other parts of a person, perhaps all of them, have a subjective conscious experience of their own, we must then distinguish consciousness from executive control. In fact, it is this issue which is posed most effectively in E.R. Hilgard's research uncovering the hidden observer, who in hypnosis is fully conscious though not in executive control — and not conscious to the usual self.

In clinical work the principle is posed by the classic multiple personality. When asked under hypnosis what his subjective experience was like when not "out," one customarily hidden secondary personality admitted to no difference from the usual except for the impossibility, when not out, of directing and controlling body musculature and consequently behavior. Contrary to having no conscious experience, being "unconscious" is, then, more like being paralyzed — watching what is going on but unable to change it or manipulate the environment.

When we accept that our minds are organized into a complex hierarchy of systems and subsystems, the issue at hand is how executive control is determined and who or what has executive control. These issues are discussed thoroughly in Hilgard's (1977) *Divided Consciousness*. Though still unresolved, they provide food for thought, further research and treatment implications.

VERTICAL SPLITS—THE DISSOCIATIVE CONTINUUM

In contrast to classic repression, where the conscious is considered above the unconscious in levels of both development and functionality, part-selves can be separated in another way. Instead of visualizing one above the other, the selves are placed beside one another. Each comprises a hierarchy of developmental levels from the most primitive to the most advanced. In place of a repression barrier, they are separated by what Kohut (1971) and Hilgard (1977) describe as a vertical split. Hilgard terms this a dissociative or amnesic barrier, its precise definition remaining problematic. Amnesia is simply a gap in awareness or memory as experienced by any particular mental unit, entity or person. Dissociation, in the broadest sense, refers to the mechanism or combination of mechanisms by which two or more collections of mental units can be kept separate from one another—the process of creating and maintaining boundaries or vertical splits between various sectors of conscious experience.

Corresponding more closely to clinical usage than dissociation in general is dissociation proper, defined by Hilgard (1977) as a condition in which customary roles lose continuity with one another. This is similar to the definition of trance I have previously proposed, the term relevant to hypnotic behavior only for individuals where hypnotic is discontinuous from non-hypnotic. Criteria for a dissociated state in Hilgard's nomenclature require the presence of internally organized entities separated from each other by a variable one- or two-way amnesic barrier, one part or state often feeling as if "possessed" by another. Fugues, possession states and multiple personalities are seen as clear examples of dissociation proper.

Hilgard's greatest contribution has been research showing that dissociation, even at its most extreme level, underlies the essence of hypnosis. This is dissociation structurally as significant as that found in multiple personalities, only in this case it enhances health. Since it is practically impossible to separate hypnotic from non-hypnotic without absurdity, even dissociation proper contributes in some way to healthy functioning, as well as being part and parcel of neurotic states experienced as a feeling of being compelled to act in a certain way by one's phobia.

I am not certain that dissociation can be explained any better than existence, consciousness or hypnosis, possibly, like them, calling for acceptance as a basic given. That it is hardly a rare or unique state or process can be seen by examining the definition of many similar terms as used by proponents of different theories of personality. State of consciousness, schema, mood, role, system, ego state and alter-personality all refer to some level of what I have simply called a mental unit. Separated by a boundary from others, each unit has characteristic features defining its identity and finite persistence over an extended period of time.

Dissociation, then, is *the process of forming and maintaining the boundary of said unit.* In order to further understanding of this phenomenon, an examination of various designations for these mental units is in order.

Discrete "state of consciousness" (d-SoC) is defined by Tart (1975) as "a unique, dynamic pattern or configuration of psychological structures, an active system of psychological subsystems. Although the component structures/subsystems show some variation within a d-SoC, the overall pattern, the overall system properties remain recognizably the same (p. 5).''

An altered state (d-ASC) is simply a d-SoC that is "different from some baseline state of consciousness." These definitions are a mental equivalent to "dynamic steady state" in the physical sciences, which I (1977a) have referred to as a "stable instability" perpetuating itself so as to satisfy the definition of an entity. As used here, it is a mental unit of sufficient complexity to encompass other mental units of a lower level of organization. If a d-SoC does not define the entire personality, it is intended at least to denote a significantly major part or aspect of it. Following the orchestra analogy, a d-SoC and d-ASC might be analogous to separate sections such as the strings or brasses, each similar to a part-orchestra in its own right, yet part of a greater whole.

The term *schema* (plural *schemata*) is used by Piaget and his followers to denote mental units of greater or lesser scope and level. Flavell (1963) abstracts Piaget's definition of schema as "a cognitive structure which has reference to a class of similar action sequences, these sequences of necessity being strong, bounded totalities in which the constituent behavioral elements are tightly interrelated (p. 53)." These can be simple motor mental units such as infantile sucking and grasping schemata or simple sensory ones for processing incoming data. The term also includes combinations at more complex levels, like the schema involving observation of a desired object and an obstacle to its acquisition, removal of the obstacle, and use of the object. At more and more complex levels of organization, the word *schema* still denotes a complex mental unit with internal coherence, discrete from other such units.

While referring to much the same thing as a "state of mind," Horowitz (1980) emphasizes the self-organizing and self-perpetuating aspects of this schema by saying that "certain self-images and role relationship models predominate in each state; we infer that these are organizing principles which are partly responsible for the repetition of a given state over time." Implicit in this statement are the boundaries and defining features between a particular state and what is outside or in a different state.

In summarizing the relevance of systems theory to modern psychiatry, Grinker (1975) writes, "Systems and subsystems constituting hierarchies, bounded by permeable borders encasing reverberating transactions, had structure functions and integrative processes (p. 269)." A system "functions in relation to other systems. In fact, the proof or validation of a system cannot come from within, but depends on its 'purpose' in relation to another system." Grinker mentions the type of thinking to which this leads as a "respectable teleology," giving meaning to human research, which should be the goal of all science.

Although Grinker's statement is in some respects similar to earlier definitions — with implications of features defining self and other, the boundaries separating them and hierarchical levels of organization — two additional features, not entirely absent from other concepts but underscored here, are worth special mention. First is an association to Watkins' (1978) definition of existence — "existence as *impact*." In his opinion, an entity can be said to exist in a meaningful sense only when its boundaries are defined by mutual impact upon other entities. With reference to my work on existence in *That Which Is* (1977a), this clearly refers to organizational existence, that of a particular pattern, not to "ontological" existence or the basic underlying energy itself. Second is the element of "teleology" that Grinker recognizes as inherent in the word *purpose*. Any psychological system appears to have a mind, purpose, and "personality" of its own — less a mechanism than a respectable teleology.

The concepts of *role*, role theory, and role enactment in modern psychology do not actually change the defining characteristics of a mental unit, but they do carrying more of a volitional-purposeful imputation. Sarbin and Coe (1972) propose a role enactment model to describe hypnosis. The primary implication in enacting a role is that it is done "as if. . . ". If we lose sight of that "as if" element in role enactment, the process becomes reified to resemble a thing or an absolute. Sarbin and Coe emphasize, however, that role-playing is not phony or make-believe; a greater danger lies in losing sight of the as-if-ness.

On the tennis court, for example, I am behaving as if I were a tennis player. To the degree to which this role is "congruent" with myself, this role enactment makes me actually be a tennis player. "*Role* is the molar concept denoting a group of behaviors that describe a functional human action (p. 67)." This still sounds the same as other terms used to define mental units. "*Enactment* describes the carrying out of these behaviors (p. 68)." "Role enactment," then, is the complete definition of a complex unit or system, with much more connotation of volition than implied by the words "state," "system" or even "schema." The boundary implications shared with the other concepts are then elaborated further. "Role *location* is the primary cognitive activity that determines the next important step in the sequence (p. 68)." This is asking the reciprocal questions of "Who am I?" and "Who are You?" from within the perspective of each role. The implication is that sense of selfhood defined in relation to others differs depending on what role we are enacting.

In a sense, each person is a different personality depending upon the particular role he is playing. A doctor, for instance, is an entirely different personality on the dance floor than when cleaning house, sharing intimacies or arguing with a loved one, working with patients or writing a book. Though differing as a person in each of these situations, within any specific role he has a persistent type of personality constellation that would meet the criteria for definition of a complex mental unit or system. In a healthy individual these roles are compatible with one another and are usually seen as aspects of the individual's overall "personality." They are still quite discrete from one another, however.

The functionality of discrete roles for different situations lies in the economy of what is left to conscious decision-making and the advantage of division of labor, that which makes higher complex organisms more effective than a giant undifferentiated single cell of the same size. While the conscious mind or executive can control at the most only two or three simultaneous activities, the unconscious collective can take part in a potentially infinite number. To "plug into" the role of a tennis player on the court, letting appropriate behaviors simply happen, is far more effective than analyzing every move.

Gallwey (1976) illustrates this superbly with regard to tennis. He states that, when Self 1 is getting a little too arrogant and wants to do it all, it can be challenged to learn the names of all the different muscles in the body, which should do what at each moment for all the possible shots in tennis. Then it could work out a system of communication which would relay all the necessary instructions to the muscles in the split-second allowed between perception and response. Faced with the absurdity of meeting such complex demands at a purely conscious level, the conscious becomes "more humble" and better able to trust in the inherent wisdom of the inner self, as epitomized by Gallwey's concept of Self 2.

Seen in this light, the value of being able to plug into any complex role, mental unit, or psychological system with role-specific skill is clear. Skill that may have taken years to develop to its current level need not be relearned, reorganized or rethought out on every occasion. It is another way of describing common experience. Although acquiring a new complex skill requires assiduous conscious effort, it appears that over a long period of learning, when role skills have become so organized as to coalesce into a complex system or schema, behavior involving them becomes progressively more automatic.

In Gallwey's second tennis book (1976), he describes beautifully the process of conscious-unconscious cooperation within the realm of tennis, indicating clearly its relevance to life in general. (I have previously presented [1977a,b] my own elaborations upon his Self 1 and Self 2 concepts and will briefly review my current position shortly.)

Similarly, other roles as complex in their way as tennis — driving or typing, keeping personal accounts or pursuing vocational endeavors — respond productively to the conscious-unconscious cooperative process. Life is so much easier when the only conscious effort required is making a decision as to which role or system to activate.

Hilgard (1977) has raised a major question concerning how the roles of Sarbin and Coe are managed. Who is the I determining which role to play of various alternatives, choosing from the many competing at any given moment for priority? This is the same question left unanswered in one assessment of Freudian psychoanalysis, depicted in my Figure 2 as the top of a pyramid with its apex up. The question concerns the nature of one's executive, discussed further below.

Hilgard's already-quoted definition of dissociation proper as a condition in which our usual roles lose continuity with one another implies — through loss of temporal continuity necessary for any mental unit — a role no longer under control of a cohesive self. Dissociation proper can then be likened to role enactment beyond voluntary control — determining, for example, to play the role of tennis player but performing instead like a cook. Behavior fully this bizarre occurs in some severely dissociated patients such as multiple personalities. That the same degree of dissociation can be and often is functional, as in hypnosis, emphasizes that we should not be too quick to put a negative value judgment on the process, however. Instead, we are advised to ask when dissociation is useful and when not.

In an attempt to clarify the terminology of *Unity and Multiplicity*, I will turn my attention first to defining the whole personality or cohesive self, then to psychological subsystems that can to a degree experience themselves in the same way. Kohut's reference (1971) to cohesive self as that which experiences itself as a mental and physical unit having extension in space and continuity in time remains in my opinion the clearest definition of selfhood. The word *experiences* is the key, leaving the concept of self free from arbitrary rigidities that could lead it into the A/Not-A absurdity. Concepts of space and time embracing the experience of selfhood, though called into question by relativistic physics, are referred to without absolutization. While selfhood as so defined often corresponds with physical boundaries of the body, Kohut recognizes that this is not necessarily so. Experience of one's cohesive self can expand beyond such limits, constrict within them, or split. It can even combine all three processes, the pertinence of each dependent upon whether it is useful or harmful.

That the experience of selfhood can vary depending upon what state a person is in at a given moment was first suggested explicitly by Federn (1952). The concept of "ego state," as defined independently and similarly by Berne (1961) and Watkins (1978), is the basis of not only transactional analysis but also any way of looking upon human behavior as a collective whole comprised of subparts, a comprehensive view not requiring adherence to any particular personality theory.

To quote Watkins (1978), an ego state is "a coherent system of behaviors and experiences with boundaries more or less permeable which separate it from other such systems within the overall Self." Berne's definition is similar. Watkins differs from Berne primarily in being less willing to fit ego states into specific categories.

Both Berne's transactional analysis and the Gestalt therapy of Perls (1969) illustrate the extent to which in normal individuals different ego states have unique personalities of their own. Classic and widely known examples involve the splitting into polar opposed states called "topdog" and "underdog" or critical parent and adapted child. Following is an illustration of Perl's topdog (T)/underdog (U) concept.

> *T.:* You lazy bum—you're doing it again! You said you'd get your room cleaned up before tomorrow, but here it is almost tomorrow. When are you going to shape up? No more procrastinating—no more "I'm sorrys." Get with it NOW, and I'm going to keep on your back until it's done.

> *U.:* You've got a good point I must admit. But remember all the things that have come up [long list presented]. I'm tired, but have good intentions. Maybe tomorrow I'll get around to it.

> *T.:* How many times have I heard that song before?

> *U.:* Well, this time I really mean it, etc., etc.

In its basic character the "alter-personality" or dissociated state, as found in diagnosed multiple personalities, does not differ from either a role or an ego state. It does differ from them in having rigid, often nearly impermeable boundaries so that there is no continuity of experience in overall selfhood when switching from one to the other. It then *seems* like an experience of two separate selves or personalities, differing from roles in being beyond voluntary control.

There is often in one alter-personality a partial or total lack of awareness of another, even of its existence, except as suggested by amnesic episodes or "blackouts" during which, the person has been told, he performed complex activities in an atypical manner. Hidden observers in hypnosis may be structurally identical to alter-personalities.

Watkins clarifies and emphasizes that dissociation is not an either/ or phenomenon, but exists along what I refer to as the *dissociative continuum*. At the simplest level of common experience are fluctuations in mood, interpreted as a state of mind organized around a particular emotion. Whether the emotion is caused by the associated ideas or vice versa is often difficult to determine. At a more intense level are the roles and ego states within which individuals perform state-specific tasks and life activities. I do not see much difference between a role and an ego state, both valid and often interchangeable, except for the connotation the terms carry, the former implying more voluntary choice, the latter existing as more of an entity. At the extreme end of the dissociative continuum are the alter-personalities or dissociated parts perceiving themselves as separate cohesive selves, as defined by Kohut.

I am well aware that this discussion on vertical splitting and the continuum of dissociation explains nothing. This is my intent. Convinced that we do not yet have precise explanations, I fear that premature attempts at precision could rigidify theories to the point of blinding us to contradictory behavior which, if recognized and dealt with competently, could be helpful in treating a particular patient as he really is — an individual whose internal organization of subparts, his "psychic politics" (Roberts, 1976), is unique.

Clarifying the many definitions of these similar terms widely in use shows the extent to which, even without actually explaining division into mental units, the phenomenon of dissociation is recognized and labeled by nearly everyone in psychology and mental health professions. I rest content to accept it in its many levels as a basic fact of life, working with this assumption and making the most of it.

THE THREE SELVES

Gallwey (1976) has presented one of the clearest descriptions of multilevel functioning in everyday life. I have already (1977a,b) abstracted his concepts of Self 1 and Self 2, relating Self 1 to the usual conscious self, an executive or conductor presiding over the personality but not actually making the music *per se*. Self 2, sufficiently personified to permit one to talk to himself, is that aspect of consciousness usually experienced as unconscious, its actions appearing automatic, involuntary, or as if just happening. I have defined Self 3 as the conscious experience of our basic biology, and described it as our link with that which is beyond, or That Which Is. It can also be defined as the experience of our *basic being*.

THE CONDUCTOR-ORCHESTRA ANALOGY REVISITED

If Self 1 is the conductor, Self 2 is the orchestra. Clearly a multiple personality in itself, Self 2 is an aggregate of lesser personalities, analogous to the various sections of the orchestra, or roles and ego states in a human being. These are themselves composed of still more personalities, the orchestra members, or the simpler schemata organized in various ways to comprise the usual self.

Here is a clear analogy to the hierarchical systems described by various theorists. Lowen (1975), for example, uses a model similar to the conductor-orchestra, that of a military general and his troops, labeling the executive "ego" and the energetics or troops "body." This may be helpful in understanding the writings of certain therapists using the term *body* in a somewhat idiosyncratic way when discussing what it wants or says. "Language of the body" is synonymous here with that of the unconscious as most hypnotists use the term.

Erickson (1976) supported my contention that Self 1 and Self 2, interpreted as conductor and orchestra, are analogous to the way he used the terms conscious and unconscious in instances when things are going "as they should." By this he meant that each part must know its own most appropriate role, fulfill it to the hilt and not attempt to usurp roles performed better by some other part of the personality. The conductor should properly be the one who conducts best, limiting himself to quality conducting and resisting any temptation to snatch the first violinist's instrument and play it whenever a bit uptight about the performance. Similarly, horn players should stick to good horn playing, respecting the conductor's role as organizer and not competing with the strings to see who can play the loudest or with the conductor to set a different tempo.

My experience with small groups or organizations of people suggests a relationship between the executive and the whole remarkably consistent for those groups functioning best as a cohesive whole — joyously, spontaneously and effectively in a disciplined manner. Without exception, the executive leader has been sufficiently strong that his authority is questioned by virtually nobody. Everyone knows who has the last word — the conductor, appealed to when trouble spots need resolution. Far from being an overcontrolling dictator, how-

ever, the leader shows a quiet strength which allows him to do less of
the work, more properly the province of group members themselves.
He sits back quietly, exerting little conscious effort, while group
members pursue their tasks enthusiastically and autonomously. The
"higher" personality of the group itself seems to just emerge, to everyone's satisfaction. Each component individual's role is so congruent
that he is truly doing his own thing, in a way that complements everyone else's. The orchestra performs by itself, the strong conductor doing little beyond providing gentle guidance at occasional trouble
spots or calling upon a certain orchestra member or section he wants
active at a particular moment.

I believe ideal intrapsychic politics are similar. The executive within, however structured, is strong and benign, feeling no need by virtue
of his strength to bully the rest of the personality. Thus, through respectful treatment of the rest he gains that respect needed for continuing effective leadership.

A clear description of things not going as they should, at a level to
which all can relate, is given by Gallwey, which I will paraphrase. The
tennis player on the court may be talking with himself. "No!—Higher,
higher, you !@#$!! idiot, when will you ever learn to—your grand-
mother could play better—now, you'd better do it right this time—
OK, now. Oh no!! dummy, you did it again!!, etc." (Here is the conductor, clearly overstepping his bounds and treating the orchestra or
inner self in a far from respectful way, but one experienced by everybody at some level.) Contrast this with being on the court, poised and
quietly confident, finding oneself, with very little sense of voluntary
effort, hitting nearly perfect shots practically inconceivable with any
amount of conscious trying.

In psychiatric practice, this analogy best fits overcontrolled obsessive-compulsive individuals who often fight themselves at considerable expense to themselves, even when they are relatively successful.
While Gallwey emphasizes the problem of overcontrol by the conscious, psychiatrists see the opposite with nearly equal frequency—a
situation in which the conductor either abdicates or is overpowered to
the extent that a variety of destructive or mad behaviors occur over
which the patient's conscious self feels he has no control. "I can't help
it—it just seems to happen."

A little imagination can suggest a nearly infinite number of ways an
orchestra could go wrong, so to speak. The string and brass sections

could be lined up behind trenches firing artillery and lobbing grenades at one another while everybody else stands by helplessly. A little prankster might set fire to the concertmaster's coattails. Someone might grab the conductor's baton, either to try conducting himself or to play "pass it around" with other orchestra members. The conductor might be lying over his podium with a bottle of whiskey while the orchestra plays chaotically, like the din of warming up before a concert. Or—and this is the most analogous to disturbed multiple personalities—the first horn player and first cellist might have batons of their own, each trying to usurp the conductor's power. Within an individual, as in social groups, things simply do not work out well when there is too much vying for executive control or when the roles of the component parts are not clearly defined and mutually acceptable.

Considering the orchestra or Self 2 (the unconscious) as a collective whole, the relationship between functions of the two parts is shown in Table 1. The terms "voluntary" and "involuntary" are as seen from the perspective of the executive, who in mental health corresponds closely to the experience of conscious selfhood. When an action is performed or decided by Self 1, it is experienced as voluntary or purposeful. When done by the orchestra without effort, it is spontaneous, involuntary and seems to just happen.

If we were to contact that part of Self 2 that actually performed an act, we would see the voluntariness at another level which in itself qualifies Table 1 as only a rough approximation of ideal function. The so-called involuntary act was actually chosen by that part, though experienced as involuntary by the usual self.

If someone (or some part) is requested to perform an act purposely, he has three options—to comply, to refuse or to do something different. Hypnotic *suggestion* is simply a request given to some part of another person that is hidden or unconscious—hence Erickson's (Beahrs, 1971) use of the term *hypnosis* as "communication with the unconscious." While the result will be experienced by Self 1 as involuntary, the same three options are present. If an unconscious part complies with the directive, the subject is said to be "responding to the suggestion" or behaving hynotically. If it refuses, he is not responding or is a "poor subject." If, as often happens in clinical hypnosis, the unconscious does something entirely different, the subject is said to be "responding in an idiosyncratic way."

Though at the executive level most healthy individuals generally

Table 1
The Three Selves

	Self 1	*Self 2*
Function	Executive (Conductor)	Energetics (Orchestra)
Level of awareness	Conscious	Unconscious
In bioenergetics	"Ego"	"Body"
Level of volition	Voluntary	Involuntary, spontaneous
To get self to do	Instruct, direct command, decide	Allow, permit, "*let* it happen"
To get someone else	Instruction	Suggestion
Type of language	Linguistic, denotative, digital	Symbolic, analogic
	Words, verbal	Behavior, nonverbal
Level of cognition	Secondary process Advanced, "higher"	Primary and tertiary process Mixed, contains primitive and "lower" along with higher
Primary in	Normal waking state	"Hypnotic trance" and some psychological states

Self 3 = Basic biology, nutrition, exercise, sleep, activity, body care
  • Spiritual Essence
  • Roots with All That Is
  • Simple Being

use secondary process or reality logic, the extent to which hypnosis involves regressed or primary process is not clear. While the unconscious or Self 2—containing the entire body of one's past learning or experience—encompasses the gamut of lower or primitive thinking mechanisms, it also contains most of the higher thought processes. As Gallwey indicates, functioning at an automatic level is often better, not worse. Arieti (1976) coined the term "tertiary process" to denote a still higher level of thinking involved in the creative process, where one has the flexibility and malleability of the primitive symbolic mode with the structure and protection of full reality logic. The best of both modes, this may be a more accurate portrayal of Self 2's way of thinking at its best.

As I have explained earlier (1977a), neither Self 1 nor Self 2 can function if not healthy. And healthy biological body functions needed for any mental unit to be at its best must definitely have a spiritual essence of their own, though perhaps at a level impossible to contemplate or put into words cognitively. Conscious experience of basic biology is what I call Self 3, the role of the body being as pertinent as those of Self 1 and all parts of Self 2 for healthy functioning. Many of the most severe mental disorders, such as psychotic depression and schizophrenia, are increasingly thought as disorders of basic biological function—genetics, biochemistry, faulty nutrition, metabolic dysfunction, or whatever.

I earlier discussed Self 3 (1977a) as the ground of being, similar to Tillich's (1951) concept of God. I conceive of it as our link with God or That Which Is. It can be seen in either its infinitesimal aspect—down to our cells, organelles, molecules, and elementary particles—or in its infinite aspect, linked in significant ways to what is outside our physical bodies and at least in principle impacting with and being impacted by everything beyond. It is easier to conceive of interacting with God in a psychological sense at primarily the infinitesimal level, this level being contained within our usual spatiotemporal boundaries. Nonetheless, it is the infinite that provides a connection with the outside world. In both we find those roots without which meaningful life would be impossible.

Figure 3 illustrates and abstracts only one of many ways in which the three selves can divide and interact, with both healthful and unhealthful consequences. It is merely illustrative. For me the beauty of the conductor-orchestra analogy is the extent to which permutations and combinations are truly infinite, encouraging us to keep our minds open to the unique combinations any difficult patient might present, unencumbered by limitations of a formal detailed theory for which we still do not have adequate data for precision.

This brings us to the issue of the central executive.

THE EXECUTIVE BRANCH OF SELF

The question of what constitutes the central executive, that intrapsychic leader who organizes and presides over the family of Self com-

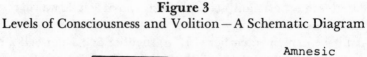

Figure 3
Levels of Consciousness and Volition — A Schematic Diagram

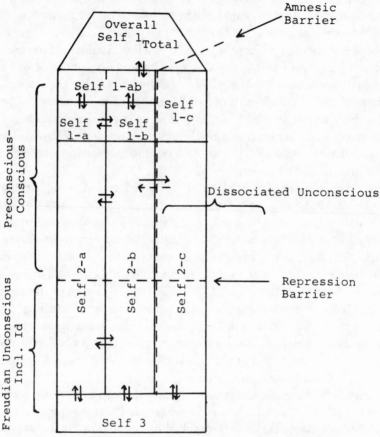

Arrows indicate flow of information.

prising a single human individual, has been posed repeatedly during this discussion. In touching upon the Freudian model in its second schematization (Figure 2), I referred to the top of the pyramid as representing the conscious, though deferring a definition. And Sarbin and Coe's (1972) role enactment model implied but did not specify a "somebody" equivalent to the conscious who chooses which role to enter and how and when.

Most pertinent, however, is the discussion just concluded indicating that if we are going to conceive of ourselves as a collective whole, we must have an organizing leader of this whole to avoid chaos. This is the job of Self 1, the conductor, his presence illustrated above and accepted as a given, though not actually defined. At the risk of sounding like a broken record, let me say that this is probably the best we can do with current data.*

That any complex organizational unit requires some executive function is practically self-evident, considering the manifold examples provided by nature, societies and even man-made machines such as computers. Yet there are two polar interpretations of the nature of the executive within the human organism. The traditional psychoanalytic one, though not held by every analyst, is that what is conscious or in executive control is determined by a hierarchy of competing systems; what is conscious is that part of the whole which at any moment has the most cathexis of psychic energy or what Watkins (1978) terms "ego cathexis." According to this point of view, there is no need to postulate an executive as a separate biological, neurological, or psychological structure.

The other polar viewpoint is to look upon someone's executive as a discrete entity in itself. Hilgard (1977) mentions the dilemma of an individual who hears the telephone ring while playing the piano. Does he continue to play the piano, i.e., stay in cognitive control system 1, or take the telephone call, switching into control system 2? The question is whether this issue is resolved by the relative strengths of systems 1 and 2, as implied by classical psychoanalytic theory, or whether it requires the decision of a central executive like a judge over and above both of them, sometimes referred to as the WILL (James, 1890).

Hilgard maintains that, if we take the former position, we are evading the problem of a planning self, the very question he raised to the role enactment model of Sarbin and Coe. "The concept of 'planning' in itself implies the concept of a planner who is doing the planning." He cites computer research as showing that even complex machines require a discrete executive who has the final say.

Hilgard also tackles the question of what gives rise to consciousness of Self, an especially tricky consideration when all parts or control sys-

---

*Hilgard (1977) presents a thorough discussion of differing viewpoints concerning cognitive control systems so clearly that I see no need to do other than refer readers interested in an in-depth discussion of where we stand at present to his *Divided Consciousness*.

tems may have simultaneous consciousness. If an inner executive is responsible for decision-making, which I personally find an increasingly unavoidable assumption, the question of what part *appears* conscious boils down to one concerning which part is actually in executive control. What the determining factor is that gives one part executive control is uncertain. A part is said to be "out" and therefore visible and apparently conscious when able to control the body's musculature. The unconscious has its own conscious experience, just hidden from the view of the part that is out, as well as from external observers.

That even this distinction is not precise is evidenced by the very datum that a hand *can* lift "by itself" as though it is "just happening" — so that the part that is "out" in the sense of being able to report its experience is not *entirely* in charge of all of the body movements. "Nonverbal" communication occurring simultaneously with verbal is a more profound and extensive illustration of this split. Three questions are then interrelated: What is the "conscious" in the usual sense of the word? Who is in charge of the body and at what level? And who carries the sense of Cohesive Selfness proper? That the answers may be different at different levels obviates the possibility of a clear and precise answer, at least with our current state of knowledge.

As I did in *That Which Is,* Hilgard emphasizes the need for a memory mechanism as the prime requisite for the sense of temporal continuity required for the experience of selfhood. There are, however, many gaps in memory, sleep being the primary one. Restoration of continuity of memory upon awakening requires a long memory store.

Observable amnesic states in which, while fully awake, one ego state does not recall behaviors and experiences of another, involve a "fractionation" of certain aspects of personality function away from the personality as a whole. Hilgard states that "if hypnosis or dissociation implies fractionation, that also implies a baseline integration from which fractionation can occur." The implication is of some centralized executive.

Hilgard's conclusions — so significant that they can no longer be taken for granted or ignored — are still admittedly not without certain unresolved ambiguities raised by his own research. Since in hypnosis executive functions shift so that what was once executive may now be hidden, there may be a split between the functions of the observing executive, which Hilgard calls the Central Monitor, and those of the active Central Executive. Yet a truly functional executive requires capabilities for both observation and action. When becoming a hidden observer in hypnosis, does the central executive merely abdicate part of his usual role, while nonetheless keeping an eye on the situation? What is the mechanism of this split within the point at the top of the pyramid? An issue raised succinctly by Hilgard himself, it demands and merits resolution.

One-way amnesic barriers are also still unexplained. Although the hidden observer in hypnosis and probably in the non-hypnotic waking state in continuity with it is aware of a subject's overtly conscious experience as well as his own, the converse is not equally true, for the subject's consciously experiencing aspect is not aware of, or is amnesic for, the hidden observer. Many secondary personalities in pathological dissociative states show the same one-way window phenomenon.

I can think of three possible mechanisms for such a split. The first, motivational, may follow if the dissociated part is disliked sufficiently by the usual self to be disowned — disowning similar to repression except that what is disowned is hidden behind a vertical instead of a horizontal barrier. This dynamic, common when an alter-personality is somewhat demonic in its behaviors, will be discussed more fully later. Here the dynamic may be collusive between the two parts, the first wanting to disown the demonic element out of fear or dislike, the second only too happy to have a screen behind which to hide while carrying out his multifarious schemes.

Another possible reason for the usual self's failure to see a hidden observer is that, wholly apart from motivation, it would be difficult to jump from one ego state to another if they were so dissimilar as to have few associational connections.

A third possible explanation is biological and awaits further brain research for elucidation. One-way amnesia is better served by the first possibility; two-way amnesia by the second. One-way amnesia as occurring in normal hypnosis is not clear. I personally prefer not to jump to any premature either/or position.

Figure 3 illustrates but one of a potentially infinite number of ways that the three selves can be divided. By subselves a and b, I am referring to the many roles or ego states that resemble subpersonalities contributing to a greater whole. They can be interchanged by voluntary choice of the overall Self 1 presented here as Self 1-ab. Each is sufficiently discrete to have some element of Self 1 and 2 of its own, subject to the higher Self 1-ab that Hilgard believes is necessary. There are many channels of communication between the two, and sufficient continuity that they are both experienced as self. Sub-Self c, denoting another role or ego state, sufficiently discordant that it is walled off or disowned behind a one-way amnesic barrier, is a *secondary personality*. Sub-Self c experiences a and b, but is not experienced by them except indirectly in the form of unwanted intrusions. Even its own Self 1-c is beyond control of the patient's usual higher Self 1-ab.

Whether there is an overall Self 1-abc or total is still open to question. Hilgard's work corroborates my own observation from professional experience that there is, though the overall Self 1-abc or Self 1-total abdicates some of its function. In that case, what can happen in hypnosis with desirable effects now becomes detrimental to the overall self. The therapeutic goal would be to restore the situation so that splitting, when it occurs, is voluntary—not a symptom but a skill.

Self 3, an individual's underlying basic biology, is assumed to be shared in common by all subselves. The horizontal dotted lines on Figure 3 refer to the repression barrier; vertical lines to dissociation barriers. Below the horizontal barrier is the repressed or Freudian unconscious, while that disowned behind the vertical barrier is the dissociated unconscious.

While I am inclined to support Hilgard's understanding of the executive branch of one's self as a separate agency and for similar reasons, I do not find the data sufficient to take an absolute position or accept it as necessarily either/or. For now I still prefer the flexibility of seeking different possibilities in any unique individual. While willfully sacrificing the specificity of a tightly worked-out theory, this approach provides more openness in perceiving an individual as he is, as opposed to what some theory indicates he "should be." Aware of assets and liabilities in either approach, I am ready to give a little, take a little and pay close attention to new research developments.

5

Dissociative Disorder— Severe, Common, Treatable

Diagnosis and treatment of dissociative disorders such as multiple personality and its equivalents provide the clinical psychiatric core of unity and multiplicity. I am focusing my discussion on multiple personality *per se* for several reasons. While true multiple personalities are by no means common, neither are they rare. Most psychiatrists have probably worked with several, whether or not they were ever diagnosed as such. This is particularly true in an inpatient setting, since multiple personalities often come to psychiatric attention in such extreme crisis as to test the limits of everyone's resources, psychotherapists as well as friends and relatives, and are often at least quasi-psychotic.

Usual diagnoses, including schizophrenia, affective disorder and psychopathy, may lead to a lifetime of chaotic misery by the very fact of not accurately addressing the issue at hand. This is especially tragic, since multiple personalities can be effectively treated. In my experience and that of most co-workers, multiple personalities are highly intelligent, creative, and well motivated. These individuals can often become pillars of society, functioning at an above average level of life fulfillment. It is always a joy to a psychiatrist when this be-

comes the case with one of his formerly most disturbed patients. I
hope this discussion may facilitate the more frequent occurrence of
such outcomes.

Multiple personality merits emphasis for another reason. It is, I
believe, an extreme caricature of processes seen in narcissistic and
borderline disorders at all levels of compensation, as well as in many
neurotic disorders—obsessional, phobic, and depressive in particular. These processes may also be seen in patients whose presenting
difficulty is substance abuse or problems with authorities. I hope and
believe that those treatment modalities definitely indicated in treatment of a true multiple personality will at some level be equally valid
for these related problems, constituting a major portion of most consulting room practice.

A unity in multiplicity approach is a new way of looking at human
problems in general. I trust the reader will extend the implications of
this discussion of multiple personality to his or her own work with different patients as they appear relevant and useful. Dissociative disorder, defined shortly, is so comprehensive a collective as to require
many volumes if I were to discuss the intricacies of applying the multiplicity framework to each psychiatric disorder. Possible applications
are therefore touched upon, but only indirectly, in my emphasis on
multiple personality *per se* as a paradigm, with the hope and confidence that each practitioner will extend the concepts in his or her own
unique way.

Further strengthening my intent to focus on multiple personality as
a paradigm is my initial statement that we are all actual multiple personalities in perhaps a more meaningful sense than the way the term is
used psychiatrically. Every individual has many internal subparts,
each with its own conscious experience, even if unperceived by his executive self and therefore relegated to the unconscious. Unlike psychiatric "multiples," however, we generally have a full experience of continuity of our selfhood. We experience our parts as exactly what they
are—parts—and our roles as what they are—roles.

The presence of ego states which may never be out in the open in no
way diminishes one's sense of selfhood. We do not have major amnesic
episodes when our behavior is not like ourselves, nor do we get into
such all-out internal wars as to paralyze meaningful life action. In

other words, the internal orchestra of a healthy individual is well ordered, unlike that of one with a dissociative disorder.

Yet, even the healthiest individuals find themselves in internal conflict at times, with episodes of disorder not unlike the dilemmas presented by psychiatric multiples, though far less severe. Thus another
reason for emphasizing multiple personality emerges in the hope of
supplying a new dimension that goes beyond psychiatry, enabling not
only the acutely disturbed, but to some degree all individuals, to re-
order their lives in increasingly productive and satisfying ways.

Use of such terms as "dissociation" and "splitting" will necessarily
remain somewhat imprecise and fuzzy, since they define a continuum
existing throughout all human life, with no discrete boundaries separating different levels or degrees of severity. We have seen dissociation
as basically the process by which one mental unit or collection of units
is set up and separated by some type of boundary from other aspects of
the psyche. These include moods, states of mind, schemata, systems,
roles and ego states, as well as alter-personalities. This unavoidable
looseness not only preserves the flexibility inherent in simplicity, but
also avoids the absurdity of defining boundaries when they are not
particularly precise in actuality.

In the most severe dissociative disorders, dissociation refers to
"when our usual roles lose continuity with one another" (Hilgard,
1977). The separated parts often conflict with each other and the flow
of information from one to the other is impaired sufficiently to disturb
the person's sense of selfhood. The distinction between different levels
of dissociation is not clear, however, and to attempt more precise distinctions than fit actual fact would lead us into the A/Not-A Absurdity already discussed.

I use the term *dissociative disorder* to denote personality splitting
that is dysfunctional, not useful or maladaptive, limiting instead of
enhancing the organism's power for action, or leading to behavior
dangerous to self and others. It refers not only to multiple personality,
but also to a broad scope of psychiatric problems where a similar dynamic applies, but with less discrete or rigid boundaries between the
part-selves. These include neurotic, borderline, and even episodically
psychotic disorders which can actually be more disturbed than true
multiples, as well as less. In apparent violation of my own principle

(1977a) that definitions should approach common usage as much as possible, my use of these two terms also differs in a significant way from common psychiatric usage because of the extent to which psychiatric usage, even if only implicitly, tends to view these processes as always pathological or not-OK.

Study of hypnosis shows that the same process at the same level can be either healthy or pathological, depending upon setting or context. That the major dissociation present even in multiple personalities is also present at some level in most, if not all, healthy humans, and may even enhance health when properly used, precludes any definition limited to negative value judgments. It is at this level of value judgment that my use of terms differs markedly from common psychiatric usage — and must. Our goal is not to be "rid" of a psychological process, but to shift it from the harmful or maladaptive ("pathological") dimension to where it is useful in its effect, so that what was once a symptom can truly become a skill.

Less severely disturbed multiple personality equivalents are those Watkins and Watkins (1979b) refer to as ego state problems. Sometimes these do not fit well into other diagnostic categories and could be treated as "mild" multiple personalities. As I use the term dissociative disorder, however, it is broad enough to encompass other clearly definable neurotic problems, including ego state problems. Seeing these other psychiatric entities also as dissociative disorders — also, not instead of — will, I hope, provide a new vehicle for easier, rapid, effective, and enduring treatment for many.

I urge the practicing psychiatrist to pay close attention to and submit to careful scrutiny the definitions of multiple personality which follow, both in the psychiatrists' current diagnostic manual (DSM-III) and as used by most experts in this subspecialty. Of equal importance will be a concise but thorough discussion of differential diagnosis (see p. 87), which I hope will result in such patients being more often recognized for who they really are, with the positive and sometimes dramatic results that can then accrue, instead of their suffering a miserable life course as "difficult patients" where nothing ever seems to fit. This may also lead to looking at other life dilemmas in new ways, within one's own working framework, that can expand potentials immeasurably in ways hard to predict.

Whether or not to work within a multiplicity framework, and if so at what level, is a decision that must be made by the practitioner on a case-by-case basis. I hope it will become clear that the issue is not whether looking upon a person as a multiple personality is "true," since we are all multiples in some sense. It is, rather, a question of whether or not this framework is useful in a particular case.

My personal belief is that such disorders not only are far more common than customarily recognized, but also raise vital philosophical treatment issues relevant to psychotherapy in general. Growing dissatisfaction with what might be called the psychotherapy ethic pervading society, along with today's increasingly stressful economic crunch, demands development of treatment methods more time- and cost-efficient that will avoid the lingering stigma of illness.

DIAGNOSIS OF MULTIPLE PERSONALITY

Criteria for diagnosing multiple personality are explicitly set forth in the American Psychiatric Association's *Diagnostic and Statistical Manual* (DSM-III): A. At any one time the individual is dominated by one of two, or more, distinct personalities. B. The personality that is dominant in consciousness at any given time determines the nature of the individual's behavior. C. Transition from one personality to another is sudden. D. Each individual personality is complex and integrated with memories, behavior patterns, and social associations. Although amnesia is mentioned as usual, it is not a defining condition.

If the definition of multiple personality set forth in DSM-III is interpreted literally, this diagnostic category will no longer be as uncommon as at present; rather, it will appear with striking frequency within both in- and outpatient psychiatric settings. This is true despite the fact that DSM-III claims this disorder is extremely rare. Not only has the looseness of the manual's definition of "personality" something to do with this, but so has its failure to define a category in which dynamics are similar but manifestations less glaring and boundaries less rigid — what Watkins and Watkins (1979b) call ego state problems. By virtue of there being no separate category for these very common disorders, they are most closely approached by the category of multiple personality.

Perhaps this is as it should be, for the similarity of treatment modalities, whether for problems of multiple personality or those of ego state, may call our collective attention to critical issues in health, diagnosis and treatment that have thus far been comparatively ignored. However, I still prefer to distinguish the more severe multiples from their equivalents. Later I will offer stricter diagnostic criteria.

My own basic position is that virtually no symptom or symptom complex and no personality type or defense is in every instance either healthy or pathological, good or evil, OK or not. I am inclined to bypass the customary implicit negative value judgments in this area along with the natural resistance to them which any person thus labeled would feel, preferring to interpret any psychological process — however detrimental it may become in the end — as originally a function or skill engaged in legitimate problem-solving. Although the problem-solving feature that originally generated the symptoms of mental disorder is often no longer appropriately employed with sufficient effectiveness to have value for either the patient or his associates, it is still a causative factor in his present debility as a multiple personality.

When considering dissociation as essential for healthy functioning, the question arises — dissociation from what? This leads naturally to the issue of cohesive self, defined by Kohut (1971) as that which experiences itself as a mental and physical unit having cohesiveness in space and continuity in time. This definition, besides embracing concepts of space and time, also implies a precise experience of self as a separate unit.

Absolute boundaries of entities, as well as absolute concepts of time and space, are, however, called into question by modern physics. The cohesive self, from which parts dissociate, may then not be so "cohesive" to begin with. Kernberg (1975) and Kohut (1971) have both defined ego-splitting as an essential feature of borderline and narcissistic personality disorders. Yet everybody has internal dialogues, a form of dissociation into subparts. Witness, for example, the common "I'm debating with myself whether to . . . ," as well as the well-known top-dog/underdog dialogues cited earlier. We have already seen the ubiquity of hidden observers.

The issue now becomes the pragmatics of: 1) When is it useful and when not to perceive oneself as a cohesive Self? 2) When as one composed of many parts? 3) And when as simply part of a greater whole? I have come to the conclusion from observation and experience that all three perspectives have a necessary place in health. Convinced as well that each can be an aspect of or even delineate what we often term psychopathology, I recognize a need to clarify more precisely when each serves a useful purpose. Even more significantly, we must delineate when each perspective is not useful, a designation I prefer to "pathological" in negating implicit value judgments and the resulting resistance I believe would follow from those.

I consider dissociation to be essential for healthy functioning; in addition, I believe that it is a creative act. Kohut (1971) has taken the same position regarding vertical splitting, which I use almost synonymously with dissociation. Everyday examples of creative dissociating are dreams and fantasies, roles and specific skills, imaginary playmates, projection of both positive and negative aspects of the self onto others, selective amnesia for stimuli, and virtually any defense function. In each, an aspect of overall mental function is put in relief by dissociation in a way that enhances one's power for action.

In defining and treating dissociative disorders, it is necessary to distinguish useful from not useful (pathological) dissociation and attempt to modify the process toward the former dimension, so that what was once a symptom becomes a skill.

DSM-III defines so limited a group of such disorders that the whole scope of the problem of unity and multiplicity is not covered. Starting with a concept of multiple personality somewhat more rigid and precise than that provided by the new manual, I have abstracted defining conditions used by those psychotherapists most active in this field to prepare a spectrum of *criteria for multiple personality:*

1) Two or more distinct personality organizations, each having a sense of cohesive selfhood as defined by Kohut (pp. 51, 66). These are generally ego states experiencing themselves as a whole or separate person and other ego states as a third person—a not-me or it. As the Watkins (1979b) so aptly put it, different ego states coexist, perceiving themselves as subjects ("me") and the others as object ("not-me"). There is variable awareness of the extent to which each is a part of a greater overall Self.

2) Amnesia. Classically, a secondary personality perceives both itself and the primary one while the primary personality or "usual self"

experiences only itself. This is similar to the relationship of the hidden observer to the experiencing self within hypnosis. While this unilaterial amnesia is approached in many cases, I have yet to see it totally achieved. Erickson (1976) shared his experience that no matter how rigid the boundaries, they are not absolute, the primary personality having some awareness of the secondary, however slight, and the secondary possibly having a degree of amnesia for the primary. Boundaries will shift from time to time, as will barriers to information exchange.

Multiples are divided by Hilgard (1977) into categories of 1) mutually cognizant; 2) those classical cases with one-way barriers; and 3) mutually non-cognizant (those with two-way barriers). In clinical experience, those are only approximations. Nonetheless, amnesia is so characteristic of the syndrome as seen in psychiatry that I would suggest that focal amnesia or repetitive blackouts (even alcoholic) with sudden personality change suggest major dissociative disorder unless proven otherwise.

3) Sudden shifts in executive control among personalities (with amnesia variable).

4) Two or more personality organizations episodically at war with one another. I include this to suggest that many multiples may never receive psychiatric attention if their part-selves are reasonably cooperative with each other.

5) Presence of the syndrome before onset of therapy. This criterion is included to negate the possibility suggested by skeptics that it is created iatrogenically to either interest or please the therapist, or by some other therapeutic artifact. This may require confirmation from ancillary sources, i.e., close friends and relatives.

Definitive diagnosis of multiple personality involves direct observation of personality changes, often with the aid of hypnosis, and communication with one or more of the alter-personalities, followed by corroboration from ancillary sources who have made similar observations. Watkins and Watkins (1979b) suggest that the major distinguishing condition from the more common ego state problems involves rigidity of boundaries and amnesic barriers—poor information exchange between the alter-personalities.

Even with criteria as rigid as those listed above, far more limiting than those of DSM-III, this condition is by no means rare. I doubt that any experienced mental health practitioner or clinic has not worked with at least a handful of multiples, whether or not they were diagnosed and treated as such.

I agree with Allison's (1977) contention that multiples are usually misdiagnosed because hypnosis, by means of which diagnosis is most easily made, is, regrettably, used by barely 10 percent of psychiatrists. Also, attitudes may reflect a negative bias toward a trait common among mental health professionals — sensitivity about our own narcissism. I also suggest that some other types of major mental disorder are overdiagnosed, often in violation of their accepted criteria. In many of these cases, a diagnosis of multiple personality not only would be more accurate, but also is necessary before the patient can have any hope of successful treatment.

DIFFERENTIAL DIAGNOSIS

Few victims of dissociative disorder have escaped the stigma of a misdiagnosis of major mental illness, which may condemn them to a stormy life within the mental health system without any significant hope of receiving the proper treatment methods, which generally do not involve use of neuroleptic drugs or lithium. In my experience the most common misdiagnoses are schizophrenia, affective disorder (manic-depressive illness), sociopathy and alcoholism with so-called alcoholic blackouts. Before I deal with these in turn, here is a hypothetical example where these differential diagnostic issues apply — commonplace in our profession.

A 30-year-old female is admitted to an acute psychiatric treatment unit in a state of terror, not being able to give a clear and coherent history of what she is worried about, but talking about such ideas as a "devil" or "demon" that is trying to take over her whole personality. She wonders whether family and friends, and perhaps the interviewer, might even be in cahoots with this devil. At times she even hears the devil's voice saying in a mocking and sneering manner, "Ah, ha, ha, your days are numbered. Why not just go ahead and kill yourself since you're not worth anything and I'm going to take over anyway" and other material similar in content. Delusions and hallucinations are present, to be sure. Is this woman schizophrenic? She probably does fit the diagnostic criteria of schizophrenia as used by most psychiatrists today, but *is* she schizophrenic?

This woman is interviewed the next day by another psychiatrist and shows no evidence of psychotic features. She gives a long history of chronic depression. While she is reasonably successful, she just does not find much spark in life and goes through her routines as a wife and businesswoman in a dull, tedious, and lifeless manner. Alarming to her, however, is that there are many gaps in her memory—she simply does not recall what transpired during these periods. She does not even remember the circumstances of her admission the preceding night or her mental state then. There is no evidence that she had been on any mind-altering drugs at that time either. She has a prior history of hospitalization for suicide attempts, but is perplexed in that she does not have any conscious recollection of having ever been suicidal or of ever having made an attempt on her life. New diagnostic dilemmas emerge. Is she simply a depressive neurotic, as her current presentation suggests? Are the amnesic episodes defensive in nature, intended to suppress or repress some highly threatening awareness? Or could she be deliberately withholding information which might get her into trouble with the authorities? If the latter is true, is she basically malingering? Was the "psychotic" episode of the night before simply part of a deliberate attempt at deception?

Additional history complicates the matter further. Review of old records indicates not only a history of acute depressive episodes with rare reference to psychosis, but also that at one time she was even diagnosed as *manic*. At that time she had been in an elevated mood, and talked with a rapid flight of ideas about rather grandiose plans for becoming active in state government and correcting many of the ills plaguing the social service programs of her state. While grandiose, and while described in a pressured and overly wordy manner, the beliefs and ambitions were not out of accord with what needed to be done and what, in fact, was not beyond the realistically possible. Is this woman an atypical manic depressive? Would she respond to lithium?

More disturbing yet, just last week a disheveled and unkempt young man knocked at her door and, when she answered, he addressed her angrily with a different name and demanded to know why she had not kept a date she had made with him three days earlier. She did not recognize this man and did not recall her activities three days earlier. What was going on? She herself said, "Am I going crazy?"

Since one of her earlier hospitalizations, she has been in ongoing treatment with a psychotherapist. She has seemed highly motivated, highly intelligent, and extremely aware of many of the issues which faced her. She seems to be a "good patient" with a high chance of success. Yet she always botches things up. After several episodes when the patient agrees to do or not to do something, violates the terms of the agreement, but tells the therapist with a straight face that she in fact has kept the agreement, the therapist wonders if the patient is actually lying. Is she a deliberate malingerer? If so, for what purpose? A survey of her legal record shows that in fact she had been arrested for a petty offense several years earlier and her sentence suspended on condition that she follow up with appropriate psychiatric treatment.

What is going on with this woman, and with the other patients who resemble her in clinical practice? At some time or another each of the following diagnoses has seemed to fit and has been applied to this troubled individual: paranoid schizophrenia, depressive neurosis, major depressive episode with suicide attempt, affective disorder, manic type, antisocial or sociopathic personality, and alcoholic. Each seems to fit the data *at a particular moment or at a particular level,* but each reduces to absurdity when one attempts to apply it to the entire picture. Instead of either-or, is it more likely either-*and?* Is she a *multiple personality?*

When a tentative diagnosis of multiple personality is made, everything fits into place and makes sense. The devil or demon by which she felt tortured was not a vague delusional abstract, but a concrete element of her own personality with which she was at war, which could be contacted and worked with by methods to be discussed in Chapters 6 and 7. Through hypnosis it was possible to activate personality segments which had been carrying out complex and purposeful activities during her periods of amnesia. One of these had made friends with the unkempt individual who had called her by a different name. Another had committed the petty legal offense and made the suicide gestures in an attempt to strike out against and possibly do away with the chronically depressed "primary" self. Another had been in executive control when she was aggressively and exuberantly pursuing her social reform ideas with such zeal that she was diagnosed as manic. In some instances the personalities seemed clearly discrete from one another, to the point of even carrying a separate name. At other times one seemed to be an aspect of the other and/or vice-versa, and the boundaries were not always clear. Nonetheless, this patient made sense and could be dealt with within a unifying framework.

Treatment was oriented toward getting each of these personalities in contact with the others, and encouraging them to communicate with one another, much in the manner of internal diplomacy. Over the course of only a couple of months, this patient made rapid progress toward becoming a healthy, creative and well-integrated member of society. There was no attempt made to fuse all of the part-selves into one great gigantic wholeness, but this seemed to happen as if by itself while things were going well. There were episodes of splitting and destructive behavior on subsequent occasions, to be sure, but none of such magnitude as to be disabling and these were always in response to a severe psychosocial stress. The patient continued to progress toward mental health.

It is not hard to see that any psychiatrist evaluating this patient at a given moment might have been led to making a diagnosis which closely approximated the mental status at any particular moment, but which did not address the overall personality. What are the criteria, if any, by which dissociative disorder can be differentiated from its many masks without the necessity of the prolonged and chaotic history which this patient endured before an accurate diagnosis of multiple personality finally made treatment possible? There are no easy and absolutely certain answers to this question, and many cases I am familiar with are still in dispute among qualified professionals. Nonetheless, I believe there are a few clinical features which can reliably differentiate the clear-cut cases of dissociative disorder from clear-cut cases of other major mental disorder with which they are often confused, bearing in mind that there is a "grey area" between different diagnostic categories (see Appendix I for discussion of psychic uncertainty).

I will now deal in turn with the diagnostic categories which we must be most careful to differentiate. In my experience these are schizophrenia, affective disorder, sociopathy, and alcoholism with blackouts — especially if they are "atypical."

1) Schizophrenia

This misdiagnosis will be made with far less frequency if we stick to the four As of Bleuler (1911), especially a pathognomonic *loosening of associations*. Bleuler considered the loosening of associations to be *the* primary disorder in true schizophrenia, from which all of the other key symptoms and signs followed as a necessary consequence. As the term "schizophrenia" is used today, even given the stamp of approval by DSM-III, the diagnosis does not absolutely require this central feature. If enough "secondary" features are presented, like delusions and hallucinations, the diagnosis of schizophrenia is considered appropriate even without the loosening of associations. I believe that this is unfortunate, and that the loosening of associations should remain the primary pathognomonic feature of schizophrenia, without which the diagnosis should be made only with grave reservations.

Even when the above patient presented with delusions of possession by the devil, and suffered the auditory hallucinations of the devil's voice, and believed that loved ones and therapist might be in cahoots with this devil, there was *no* true loosening of associations. Though delusional, she presented herself coherently, and the voices themselves presented coherently. Were loosening of associations used as a true criterion of schizophrenia, the evaluating physician even then and there would have been forced to consider the possibility of an alternative diagnosis, here multiple personality, which actually fits the data even better than paranoid schizophrenia. Loose associations, where one idea leads to another without a logical connection, is rarely present in dissociative disorders like multiple personality (even when one ego state of many may be psychotic). While multiples may hear voices, they are coherent; there may even be coherent hallucinatory dialogues between persecutory and protective voices. Patients usually talk coherently without loose associations even when psychotic.

Frequently, multiples report severe to extreme adverse reactions to all neuroleptics tried. When that history in an otherwise atypical "schizophrenic" is brought to my attention, I take it seriously. Some, failing to consider the tragic possibility of a major diagnostic error, say the absence of response to neuroleptics indicates a patient so schizophrenic as to need even more medication. May's (1968) monumental study shows that approximately 30 percent of diagnosed schizophrenics respond to psychotherapy but not to medication. Perhaps we need to take a closer look at that 30 percent.

2) Affective Disorder

Multiple personalities and their equivalents are frequently misdiagnosed as suffering from bipolar affective disorder (manic-depressive illness), especially with our profession's interest in antidepressant medication and lithium. This diagnosis is especially apt to be confused with dissociative disorder, because the very nature of the dissociative process involves splitting into discrete segments of self which are often manifest in nearly opposite and contradictory ways. Frequently, a primary personality is chronically depressed, having access only to a small portion of the patient's overall life energy. A secondary personality, having access to most of this split-off energy, may at times take over executive control and behavior in such an overexuberant and uncontrolled fashion as to warrant a descriptive diagnosis of mania. Rare is a multiple personality for whom a diagnosis of bipolar affective disorder has not at least been given serious consideration, if not employed. This is as it should be, since it is just as tragic to miss a diagnosis of a patient who will respond to lithium treatment as it is to miss a multiple personality such as the case above. We do, however, need to be aware that patients presenting with wide mood swings are not automatically affective disorders, and the dynamic may be entirely different. If two or more coexisting parts of the personality are of different extreme moods, of what value would be the giving of an antidepressant? While it is often difficult to resolve this dilemma for any given patient, I believe there are some guidelines.

Multiples misdiagnosed as manic-depressive do not demonstrate the true cyclicity of the latter disorder, nor do they respond to lithium therapy. Personality changes are so sudden, dramatic and unpredictable, yet so understandable when the dynamics are on the table, as not to fit the biological paradigm of the affective disorders. The shifts from manic to depressed states may occur within hours, minutes or instants; they rarely take place over days as is characteristic of true affective disorder.

This diagnosis is often made in multiples because at least one alter-personality may show such boundless energy, grandiosity and poor judgment as to suggest a true manic state. Further complicating matters is the fact that some true manics will be amnesic for their highs, even with the diagnosis confirmed by complete and enduring remission with lithium treatment. It is the suddenness of the transitions, usually with amnesia, that gives the clue. Long-term absence of response to medication also suggests that we take a closer look. At times, a multiple personality treated with lithium will show signs of lithium toxicity at or even below low therapeutic range. As is the case with schizophrenia, poor or even highly adverse reactions to the usual medications of choice should strongly suggest that we take a second look at the original diagnosis and consider alternate possibilities.

Schizophrenia and affective disorder are the two major categories which at times must be ruled out in the diagnosis of dissociative disorder. As with any medical or psychiatric disorder, there can be elements of both and a grey area in between, but at least in principle the categories can at times be either/or. This is not so clearly the case in the differential diagnoses which follow. First, with sociopathy, and then even more with alcoholism and neurotic and borderline disorders, the differential diagnosis is not either-or but either-*and*. Increasingly, the alternative diagnosis is not presented as "instead of," but is equally accurate "in addition to." The boundary between deliberate misinformation (sociopathy) and involuntary amnesia (multiple personality) is so blurred, and the consequences so profound in court of law that a notorious case history is presented in depth as Appendix II. Further, major dissociation is simply another way in which unquestionably diagnosed alcoholics, neurotics, and borderlines can be conceptualized and treated.

3) Sociopathy

The incongruity in statements made by one ego state as opposed to another often suggests intentional lying. Deliberate faking or "conning" is the usual counter made by the prosecution to cases in which multiple personality has been used as a defense in court. This is especially interesting in that the dissociative syndrome may have originated during childhood by exactly such a con—for example, "I didn't do it—Johnny did." When this is done enough under sufficient duress, "Johnny" may assume a personality with his own separate experience (Hawksworth and Schwarz, 1977). Perhaps nowhere else in psychiatry do we have a clearer demonstration of the *decisional* model presiding over the medical, with affective disorders being at the other extreme.

Most of the characteristic features of the sociopath (a consistent lifelong pattern of delinquent behavior) are absent in the multiple. We simply have the incongruity, often as unfathomable to the patient himself as to those so ready to label and mislabel. I have worked with a transitional case who could be called a "two-and-a-half personality." Her primary "usual self" will sometimes willfully withhold information about undesirable behavior to avoid disapproval. While this is true conning, it sometimes escapes the patient's awareness and voluntary control, at which times she also "cons" herself, an alter-personality being one representative of what is disowned by this process.

4) Alcoholism

Many alcohol abusers reach a stage where they suffer blackouts or prolonged amnesic episodes, during which they behave in a danger-ous and abusive manner, as if a different person. Upon close question-ing of these patients, I find that most can recall at least one similar episode occurring while sober. Also, I have personally known too many individuals who can drink themselves into oblivion socially without anything remotely suggestive of a dissociative episode.

Alcohol may be more of a facilitator than a cause of the underlying "personality" that gets "let out." Alcohol intoxication is one of two methods *par excellence* for letting out a persecutory alter-personality. The other is hypnosis, which is therapeutic in providing more rather than less control. It is likely that in many alcoholics the substance abuse is secondary to a primary dissociative disorder.

5) The "Difficult Patient"

Multiples frequently present with severe chaotic psychopathology in an otherwise successful and productive individual, challenging the resources of the most skilled therapists. They are appropriately desig-nated "difficult patients" — nothing seems to fit or make sense and nothing works that should. Transactional analysts may describe these patients as having a third degree "don't be" script, because despite their overall success they always seem to do something to bring them back to the bottom. Yet when a dissociative syndrome is diagnosed, everything seems to fall in place, with therapy usually progressing rapidly.

In summary, any major persisting and seemingly unfathomable *incongruity* should suggest that we keep a high index of suspicion for major dissociative disorder. In regard to the designation of difficult patient, I recall Braun's (1979) caution to prospective therapists that after facing this problem, "You will never be the same."

TYPES OF DISSOCIATIVE DISORDER
AND THEIR EQUIVALENTS

1) *Multiple personality*—a paradigm, already defined.

2) *Ego state disorders* (per Watkins and Watkins, 1979a, b), a category needed only when the most rigid criteria for true multiple personality are employed. This group consists of those patients with virtually the same dynamics and diagnostic features as multiple personalities, but with all aspects less rigid and blatant. Amnesic barriers are looser and variably permeable, and there is a variable awareness on the part of most, if not all, subparts that this is what they are—only parts. Each part nonetheless has its own subjective experience, often wanting to become a separate person and to be rid of other part-selves. Diagnostic features and indices of suspicion are the same as for multiple personality. Frequent expression of the desire to get "rid of" some ill-defined aspect of one's self suggests taking a closer look at what it is the patient wants to rid himself of—often a valid collection of behaviors and experiences with at least a partial sense of its own identity.

The following can all be classified as among ego state disorders. Where another diagnosis is appropriate, it is not a manner of either/or but either/and. Whether to use an explicit formulation of ego state disorder depends on the utility of doing so. I would use the term *ego state disorder* as a primary diagnosis only in cases for whom the basic dynamics of multiple personality apply in less blatant form, and where alternative diagnoses cannot be employed without risk of misinformation. I differentiate ego state disorder from true multiple personality primarily on the basis of one criterion: In the former, there is no sense of discontinuity of actual selfhood. Each subpart or "personality," no matter how discrete and different, is still experienced as an aspect of an overall cohesive selfhood, not *as if* it were a separate self as the case in true multiples.

a) *Nominalizations ("Its") Experienced as Persecutory,* of which the patient feels himself the victim. In neurotic disorders, a compulsion, phobia, or agitation is perceived as an "it," which comprises practically the full extent of the patient's usual subjective experience of what is, in actuality, a vast and well-organized pool of psychic energy. Often this has personality features of its own and ordinarily it has full awareness of itself, as well as of the patient's usual experience. Here is the same one-way amnesic barrier we have referred to before, just at a less extreme level than in full-blown multiple personality. Bandler and Grinder (1975) refer to this as a nominalization, Sullivan (1953) as a not-me.

Gestalt techniques described by Perls (1969) demonstrate that hidden personality elements can easily be re-accessed, and I earlier described use of similar techniques in a hypnotic context (Beahrs and Humiston, 1974). Even within conventional psychotherapy, techniques necessary for treating multiples can often be employed successfully as optional facilitators.

b) *Internal Dialogues* are universal in human experience. The most common example, often dysfunctional, is what Perls terms "top-dog-underdog," or Critical Parent vs. Adapted Child. Whether or not internal dialogue is functional depends on cooperative give and take, subject to control of the central executive. This is also true for all major dissociation and is a precondition of health. Orchestra members work together cooperatively under the leadership of the conductor. When communication becomes an internal war, it may lead to the paralysis of inaction characterizing many depressed and compulsive individuals.

c) *Borderline Syndrome.* Kernberg (1975) and Kohut (1971) describe major ego splitting as characteristic of narcissistic and borderline personality disorders. Although in borderlines the splitting may be too chaotic to form stable personality organizations as in multiples, this has not been my usual experience. As long as schizophrenic loosening of associations is not a factor, stable subpersonalities are there and can be found, often at war with one another. There may be an intricate system of partial and total amnesic barriers giving the appearance of chaos. And chaotic and unfathomable disturbances in an otherwise healthy individual are the hallmark of dissociative disorder. I do not believe the two are necessarily separate.

Gruenewald (1977) maintains — and I could not agree more — that multiple personality falls into the rubric of narcissistic and borderline disorders, as opposed to the hysterical. What is a multiple personality if not a disorder of self, the essence of the narcissistic dilemma? Reviewing DSM-III, I have difficulty finding any multiple personalities who do not also fit the criteria for borderline syndrome. With the new manual's encouragement of multiple labels when needed for accuracy, the proper diagnosis is then "Borderline Personality Disorder with Multiple Personality." I am not certain to what extent the converse applies regarding the percentage of borderlines who are also multiples. With the loosened criteria for multiple personality, now including ego state disorders as well, I suspect the percentage is great.

ETIOLOGY

The etiology of dissociative disorder is as poorly understood as the phenomenon itself. I refer again and again to Kohut's (1971) statement about vertical splitting, that it is a creative act or choice of the organism designed to enhance its power for action or to defend against some threat. This skill can be employed in a useful or maladaptive manner. In discussing psychiatric patients one must assume the latter, that the skill is not working to the organism's advantage; otherwise he would not be presenting as a patient.

What is the basic skill to begin with? Hilgard (1968) has argued convincingly that individuals vary in their ability to experience hypnosis in controlled conditions. That hypnosis is also a dissociative phenomenon would suggest that capacity for creative dissociation also varies from person to person and parallels what is loosely termed hypnotizability. In the same (adverse) environmental conditions, why does one individual develop a schizophrenic disorder, while another develops an obsessional neurosis or a character disorder? And why do still others become multiple personalities? The last, I suspect, are those who have the requisite hypnotic skill to begin with. Supporting this contention is the observation that virtually all multiples either are or can become virtuoso hypnotic subjects.

The basic purpose of all such symptoms was originally either to protect the self or to enhance power for action. In what ways can this go wrong? There appear to be many roads to a split personality:

1) *Avoiding Mental Friction* (Watkins, 1979). If an individual has large areas of personal need and satisfaction in one area experienced as incompatible with satisfaction in another, there is a likelihood of conflict and anxiety. The role of this circumstance in neurotic disorder was well described by Freud (1916). If areas of need can be separated or dissociated from one another and allowed to "slip by" each other with comparatively little contact, friction or anxiety is reduced. Watkins uses the analogy of a man who has a wife at one end of town and a mistress at another, making sure there is plenty of distance between them so as to minimize conflict. Within a particular individual the advantage is clearly avoidance of conflict and anxiety—for a while. The disadvantage, which may not catch up with him until much later, arises from the decrement in information exchange between the two parts, which may become the well-known amnesic barrier. Contradictory behavior in the outside world then leads to the real-life external conflicts which are legendary among multiple personalities.

2) *Imaginary Playmates.* Pines (1978) has demonstrated that children who create imaginary playmates are generally healthier and more adaptable than those who do not. Kampman (1976) has demonstrated that highly hypnotizable subjects capable of creating multiple personality syndromes upon suggestion are likewise more adaptable than those who cannot. However, Congden, Hain, and Stevenson (1965) have reported a well-documented case of transition from an imaginary playmate to a maladaptive alter-personality. The pathology most likely arises when the playmate is invested with so much ego cathexis (Watkins, 1978) that it assumes a subjective experience of its own. Even then, problems do not necessarily ensue unless the characteristics are so negative to the overall self that the playmate is disowned, again hidden behind an amnesic barrier. Only then does an individual lose both information exchange and control, resulting, all too frequently in war between the two parts.

3) *Escape from Responsibility.* A childhood version of "not guilty by reason of insanity" and an outgrowth of the above is an attempt to

avoid punishment by saying, in essence, "I didn't do it—Johnny did" (Hawksworth and Schwarz, 1977). If this is said often enough, the child may actually believe it; "Johnny" is then isolated from consciousness behind an amnesic barrier. He is imbued with the qualities most likely to invoke punishment, suggesting in itself that he will be negative in most of his behavior. When this primitive alter-personality still exhibits behaviors not acceptable as an adult, but is unrecognized by the patient in his usual personality state, is that person then really criminally insane? Several such cases have been tried, the verdict going both ways. Loss of voluntary control is definitely a feature of the clinical syndrome; further, the alter-personality over which control is lost is not only hidden beyond an amnesic barrier but may often be so primitive as not to realize the nature and consequences of its actions in the sense required for legal responsibility. The issues are far from simple.

4) *Amnesia and Abdication of Control.* Probably the cardinal distinguishing features between dysfunctional splitting and health, amnesic barriers can occur either suddenly or gradually, as confirmed by both clinical data and hypnosis research. Detailed understanding of the mechanism awaits further research.

5) *Hypnotic Negation of Sense of Self.* Harriman (1943) has demonstrated that when a responsive, normal hypnotic subject responds to a suggestion which negates his sense of self, an alter-personality spontaneously emerges. This illustrates another possible mechanism by which the clinical syndrome may originate. Children of the age where major dissociating usually occurs are almost universally responsive hypnotic subjects, whether or not they continue to be in later adult life.

It is well-known that the environment from which multiples grow is often hostile and sadistically punitive, and that double-binds are imposed with a demonic vengefulness. The child will almost always perceive extreme "Don't be!" messages. One way of coping with these might be to stop existing symbolically, by an autohypnotic (imaginative) choice to negate his sense of being. As with Harriman's study, alter-personalities may then emerge spontaneously. I believe this merits further study.

6) *Environmental Factors and Developmental History.* Most prevalent in the early life environment of the multiple is the all-pervasive

incongruity. Parents and authority figures themselves said and did
one thing, while saying and doing another on a different level. One
patient may deal with incongruities or double-binds by going crazy,
another (healthier) by leaving the environment, and yet another by
creating his own incongruity to match that of his environment.
Given the basic hypnotic or dissociative ability I consider a prerequisite, splitting will more likely lead to a multiple personality syndrome or its equivalent.

Traumatic episodes, both single and multiple, are often identifiable in the backgrounds of multiple personalities. Incestual rape
is common in the history of female multiples, gross physical abuse
in males. Often an alter-personality can specify the exact time,
place, method and purpose of its origin — usually protective, often
of life. Validating that original protective purpose may be a good
way to develop rapport with an otherwise hostile ego state and is
often the initial psychotherapeutic intervention.

Stern (1980) describes two stages in the formation of a multiple personality: 1) the formation of a dissociated state and 2) its subsequent
emergence as a separate personality in its own right. These may occur
simultaneously or be separated by a gulf of many intervening years.
With normal ego states the second stage never occurs except under
hypnosis and then only transiently. Stage one may occur by the gamut
of means for the purposes already discussed — and more. It almost invariably occurs during childhood and its purpose is usually protective
of survival, enhancing power for action. Identification of the circumstances of its origin, usually by hypnotic age regression or an equivalent, helps both to clarify the purpose of a secondary personality state
and to quiet criticism that it may have been created by a therapeutic
artifact.

Emergence into observable overt behavior, stage two, may not occur until much later in life, even adulthood. The underlying processes
are again manifold. Stage two will occur whenever the dissociated
state becomes cathected with sufficient psychic energy to take over
the subject's voluntary musculature or "come out." When a secondary
personality first comes out in a therapeutic setting, either under the
stress of self-scrutiny or from therapeutic permission, the question of
artifact is of course less easy to dismiss. When this first occurs in adult-

hood in association with a criminal offense, the differential diagnosis from sociopathy becomes more difficult as well as more urgent — complicated by its not always being either/or.

Using systems theory, Calof (1979) is studying how multiple personalities, once they become overt, maintain their syndromes through interaction with their environment. Like most investigators, he sees the formation of discordant personality states as a way of coping with irreconcilable incongruities in a patient's early background. Personality state A_1 may have been an attempt to please father's ego state A; B_1 an attempt to please father when in a contradictory state B. This may have been the best possible way to live in a disturbed home, though it loses its value in the larger social structure as that individual grows up.

If he continues to shift between personalities A_1 and B_1 even when not appropriate, he can only baffle friends, therapists and authority figures. Simply being human, they respond to his incongruity with state-appropriate behavior of their own, referred to as behaviors A_2 and B_2. Since these are in response to what had themselves originally been responses to A and B, they tend to resemble those original pathogenic binds. The patient's reaction in perceiving A_2 as A, and B_2 as B is to conclude that people are simply that way, not recognizing his own role in perpetuating an undesirable and unnecessary response.

A_1 leads to A_2 which then reinforces A_1 — like much of psychopathology, a vicious circle. This circle must be kept in mind by therapists when treating difficult patients with incongruent behavior. Especially with an undiagnosed multiple, a therapist is more likely than not to perpetuate the disorder by not recognizing it for what it is, since he too will respond with his own different states to those of his patient. In the absence of open discussion of the problem, all the patient will perceive is that the therapist's behavior, "like everybody else's," is double-binding.

Most investigators agree that the earlier the chronological age at which major personality splitting occurs, the greater the number of alter-personalities the patient is subsequently to manifest. Beyond that, however, there is considerable disagreement about the relative prevalence of duality, multiplicity and super-multiplicity (my term for multiples with 20 or more identifiable alter-personality states). Allison (1979) claims that most multiple personalities are truly multiple, with more than two. Braun (1979) believes that if you look closely

enough, they often prove to be super-multiples. Both would agree
that circumscribed dual personalities develop only when the primary
split occurs relatively late in childhood or during early adolescence.
Supporting their clinical observation, they reason that further splitting is nearly inevitable, the patient having demonstrated that dissociation is his major defense in difficult situations, one which even his
alter-personalities will continue to use throughout life, with new
alter-personalities the result.

My own experience differs, as does that of Watkins and Watkins
(1980). I have diagnosed close to ten clear-cut dual personalities, but
only a few multiples with three or more identifiable part personalities,
and no super-multiples. This does not mean that I have never worked
with a super-multiple, any more than the fact that those psychiatrists
not believing in dissociative disorder have never worked with a multiple means that multiples do not exist among their patients. It does
mean that so far it has not proved useful to me to look for more personalities than parsimoniously makes sense of the patient's problems
in living.

I am not certain to what degree this explains contradictory data regarding duality versus multiplicity, in which I differ from many respected colleagues such as Allison and Braun. Most likely it is a matter
of their describing as an additional personality or two in multiples
what I would describe as simply an aspect or facet of either the primary or secondary personality, preferring to keep as simple a perspective as possible. While these patients have truly demonstrated their
ability at splitting, it is also well to keep in mind that the major pathogenic splits may have occurred only under the most extreme stress. It
is possible even for them that at other times those synthesizing and
organizing forces of the mind that give most people their sense of cohesive selfhood might hold sway. "Once a multiple, always a super-
multiple" does not take into account all the variables.

The inevitable question then arises: Why not simplify still further
by defining only a single personality or Self, the position of most psychiatrists? Bearing in mind that we are all not only one, but, despite
subjective experience, also split into many subparts or ego states, as
well as being part of a greater whole, makes the issue not one of truth
but of what is mose useful. If and when the splitting is so severe as to
have two or more parts at war, with separate subjective experiences

and amnesic barriers, I see no way to avoid calling a spade a spade and dealing with the individual as a true multiple, which includes talking as a therapist to different part-selves as if they were truly separate individuals. In one memorable case, I had to deal with 12 distinct personalities. In none have I found any value in looking for and finding as many as 20 or 30, as does Braun (1979). I am well aware also that the answers are not yet in.

I would not be at all surprised if a close study of severely disturbed borderline patients, those I often look upon as splitting in too chaotic a manner to form stable alter-personalities, might reveal that they approximate Braun's (1979, 1980) super-multiplicity. If that is the case, treatment of collections of part-selves as a single multiple personality might precede work with the fewer number of more integrated part-selves that we would then be left with, proceeding toward integration in reverse order from the fragmentation which originally occurred. This is indeed close to a summary statement of Braun's methodology as I understand it.

The above becomes too much like hard work, however, as Braun himself readily acknowledges. Following the criterion of what is *useful*, I am not yet convinced of the utility of seeking out, finding and working with as many as 40 separate personality states. Treatment would then become virtually as lengthy and demanding as the psychoanalytic methods propounded by Kohut (1971) which I hope the multiplicity model might short-cut.

It is interesting to consider that in highly creative individuals who nonetheless present with many of the features of the narcissistic or borderline personality disorder, the "defect" may not be any defect at all in absolute terms. If the conductor is as strong in absolute terms as any normal individual but the different orchestra sections are stronger, then the conductor will be weaker *relative to* the orchestra sections and the same type of symptomatology might manifest but at a different level. That there is at least a loose correlation between dissociative skill and intelligence is suggested by the fact that intelligence itself refers to problem-solving ability which to a large degree is dependent upon a person's ability at breaking things down into categories and then logically manipulating these categories — a reframing of dissociation as increasing one's power for action by means of division of labor.

An extremely intelligent individual might develop himself to a high level of achievement in many different areas of life and may separate his roles within one sphere of living from another to the degree that they are almost as if separate personalities, even though they are clearly aspects of him. Let us consider the possibility that this intelligent person might have an organizing force or conductor of approximately the same strength in absolute terms as an individual less creative and intelligent. If this individual's subparts are themselves so much more highly organized and strong in themselves than those of the average person, then his executive would be weaker *relative to* his subparts, compared to the normal individual. From this might arise an individual structurally similar in many ways to features seen in narcissistic and borderline disorders, though functioning at very high levels.

I wonder, to what extent this might apply to many well-known historical figures who have achieved the highest levels of creativity but were never able to transcend highly disordered and conflicted personal and social living. A classical example would be Richard Wagner, whose Ring cycle portrayed a unique awareness and understanding of the polarities and paradoxes of human life to a degree almost unparalleled in human literature (Donington, 1963); yet he was unable to order his own chaotic and at times very disturbed life.

Clinical support for the multiplicity model is primarily pragmatic. It has the potential to set forth in clear relief the relevant issues for a given patient in such a way that treatment can be abbreviated dramatically in both time and effort. This holds true for dual and low-degree multiple personalities, as well as for those more fragmented multiples for whom a few common denominators can be found. When we go too far toward super-multiplicity, the usefulness dissipates, the main support for the position of multiplicity losing force. It is here that we can say the limits of relevance of the multiplicity approach have been passed.

Some indirect encouragement for a low-degree multiplicity approach was given by a former patient whom I had successfully treated as a dual personality. When functioning as an integrated person, he was able to report an awareness of five distinct alter-personalities, all dating back to childhood. These had come together successfully without having been dealt with separately by the therapist. It is not always necessary, then, to identify and work with every tiny piece that has its own experience to make healthy living possible again. What had been necessary in the professional setting was that the dissociated element most discordant to the personality as a whole be welcomed back into the family of Self, at which time other less discordant personality fragments could be dealt with by the now stronger patient without therapeutic intervention. And this most discordant secondary personality which I worked with had sufficient facets to his own personality that whether or not to call him a multiple within was not necessarily relevant. I hope that this sort of process may eventually prove workable with the more highly fragmented borderline individuals.

Splitting seems to caricature the good/evil dichotomy, with the secondary personality (not-me most of the time) showing characteristics appearing evil to the patient in his usual states. Hence, these aspects of himself are disowned. If cathected with sufficient psychic energy, this is at a heavy price, since the patient fails to rid himself of aspects to be disowned, merely pushing them out of awareness. First banished by the patient's conscious choice, these aspects of selfhood may then hide or are hidden behind an amnesic barrier. Since the disowned aspects are generally those which an individual would not like exposed for public any more than private view, it is not difficult to see that the resulting alter-personality might have undesirable traits. For the stress to have required disowning in the first place, there is probably considerable psychic energy invested in the disowned part-self.

Result? The usual self we are left with is often a rather empty, lifeless, but morally straight "goody-goody" who tries to help others and generally gets pushed around in the process. But the life energy he had disowned has hardly disappeared. In those we diagnose as multiple personalities, the associated personality aspects that are disowned smoulder under or beside the surface and coalesce into what experiences itself as a cohesive self of its own, often without its being aware that it is actually but a part-self. Since this personality does not appreciate being kept under a lid or paralyzed, it may take whatever opportunity presents to come out and in a rage deliberately disport itself with virtually no behavior controls, getting the primary personality — now the not-me — into trouble. This describes dual personality in its most typical presenting form and illustrates a most common type of dysfunctional alter-personality, a "persecutor."

TYPES OF ALTER-PERSONALITIES

Allison (1977) classifies alter-personalities as seen in major dissociative disorders into three different categories—persecutors, rescuers, and internal self-helpers (or ISHs). The first two are considered pathological, the last a healthy personification of the creative unconscious which we all share.

Most common in clinical practice is a *persecutor,* since by definition this is an ego state that gets the self and others into trouble, rendering clinical attention all the more likely. Though there are as many kinds of persecutors as human individuals, no two alike in all regards, I have found just two major types in my clinical experience.

First and most common is that personifying the large body of a person's life energy after it has been disowned, then turning upon itself in rage. The formation of such persecutors is probably similar to Sullivan's (1953) not-me and Lowen's (1967) demons and monsters.

Demon, a commonly used term for what often ensues, is usage I will adhere to while making it abundantly clear that I do not share the dislike of demons that leads to suppressing and angering them. A demon has seemingly boundless energy, which leads to many multiples' being misdiagnosed as manic. A pure demon, when fully free and out, may like to have fun with little or no behavior control, often at the expense of the primary personality.

While disaster and atrocity may be their handiwork, demons are clearly not evil in their basic being, as I hope to illustrate with a case summary and discussion in Chapter 7. They personify pure life energy, with undesirable effects only when misdirected.

More than anywhere else in psychiatry, demons raise the paradoxes inherent in good and evil. When the life energy functions of a demon are validated and accepted by the overall Self, the demon may quickly change from a seeming enemy into the individual's greatest asset. He recognizes that the problems ensuing from inadequate behavior control endanger himself as well as his "host" and out of sheer joy of living may welcome sufficient restraint from without to make continuation of life more likely. The demon may now enjoy the protection provided by the primary personality's moral structure, while the latter enjoys the infusion of vital life energy formerly disowned. Whenever this is a slow process, the difficulty is less likely reluctance on the demon's part than resistance of the primary personality, arising from fear.

A second type of persecutor is rarely seen as a full-blown alter-personality; I have seen only one so far. It is common, however, in ego state problems and their neurotic equivalents. To the degree that it is apparent in rigid personalities, I call this persecutor a *tyrant*. This seems better terminology than Steiner's Pig (1979) or my alternative designation, Bully, though they denote substantially the same. This particular persecutor acts more like a compulsive and stiflingly critical parent, torturing his "victim" with overweening directives that cannot be satisfied and then bullying him with "don't be" messages. Appearing to lack the life energy of a demon and to be as depressed as their victims, tyrants may be particularly difficult to work with. Validating that part's underlying fear and providing protection works best, though that is easier said than done in actual fact.

Watkins (1980) describes what could be considered a variant of the demon or even a wholly different type of persecutor. If considered a third type, I would label it an *avenger*. In settings where expression of anger is forbidden, though a feeling of anger is unavoidable, especially in homes where a child is the subject of recurrent sadistic brutality, the child may first create an imaginary playmate as an escape. While seeing this new entity as object, he may project all his rage onto it so that he can disown it and escape the consequences of his rage.

As this object becomes increasingly loaded, the child walls it off more and more until it is hidden behind a dissociative barrier, loaded with all that rage projected upon it. With a shift from what Watkins (1978) calls object cathexis to subject cathexis, this ego state assumes its own personality and, now perceiving the original subject as object, vents its wrath.

Some notorious homicide cases may illustrate this dynamic. Fortunately these extreme cases are rare, though notorious enough to capture public attention and feed a fear of dissociative problems. Since I have worked with few patients of this type, I do not know to what extent they can benefit from the same treatment paradigm as a demon. Unfortunately, what the avenger avenges is rarely its rightful target and even then it is destructive to all concerned.

Whether or not we need to distinguish Watkins' two types of cathexis, subject and object, is uncertain. If we accept the position of simultaneous co-consciousness, both have a simultaneous experience of self as subject and other as object. The avenger probably had some subjective experience of his own from the moment he was created as an imaginary playmate. He only became more estranged the more he was separated from the rest of the self and increasingly powerful the more he was invested with psychic energy. Having always regarded the rest of his self as object, the switch when he took over may not have been so much in subjective awareness as in executive control. When he became able to control the muscles and impact the environment, nobody could then fail to take notice—within or without his overall self.

Another major type of alter-personality described by Allison (1977) is a *rescuer*. In a multiple personality a rescuer may be created to offset a persecutor, the two possibly forming a pair of seeming opposites like a topdog and underdog. In his usual state the patient may hear coherent voices of persecutor and rescuer in dialogue.

An example of a "rescuer" is a part-self whose overall attitude is "let's make the world a wonderful place to live." When in charge of the person's body, the rescuer may attempt to "make things wonderful" by obsequiously placating behavior toward other individuals which almost always meets a response of disgust, avoidance, or anger. It might involve turning the other cheek in a manner that does not paralyze another individual with love, but is more likely to invite a retaliatory blow for something that another part-self has just done. In the social sphere it might be similar to Neville Chamberlain's encouragement of Hitler's abuses by rewarding them. At best, it would be that which runs the risk of bad consequences for behavior which was done in goodwill but with hideously poor judgment. Like persecutors, rescuers are child ego states and their defective judgment is a reflection of the immature level of cognition usually characteristic of the stage at which these part-selves were formed. As with persecutors, treatment is oriented toward validating the positive purposes of these parts and helping them function even more positively in a more effective and appropriate manner.

Steiner (1971) defines "rescuing" in a pathological context as doing for someone what he could better do himself. Karpman (1968) describes a "Drama Triangle" with three pathological positions, seemingly different but each a variant of the same, as evidenced by rapid switches from one pole to another. These are victim, persecutor and rescuer. When the victim realizes he is no better off for the "rescue," he may become persecutor to the rescuer, switching the latter to victim. The same type of dynamic can be observed within a given personality in some multiples. Rescuers are a problem clinically only when they become persecutors or bind energy which should be made available to the rest of the personality.

Set apart from "pathological" alter-personalities are what Allison terms *internal self-helpers* or ISHs. He reported a case (1974) in which an ISH had emerged spontaneously during treatment and assumed the role of primary therapist, the psychotherapy then progressing rapidly toward a satisfactory resolution. This led Allison to explore the ISH phenomenon in depth, concluding that internal self-helpers are present in all multiples, have characteristics differing from pathological alter-personalities and are probably the greatest resource for treatment. In his view, they differ in having 1) no identifiable time and reason for their formation; 2) no defensive function; and 3) far more accuracy of perception, to the point of being "incapable of transference" and able to tell a therapist all his mistakes. Watkins, Allison and I see the ISH as comparable to Hilgard's hidden observer in normal hypnotized subjects; Braun (1979) further notes that there may be many ISHs.

Allison (1977) describes a hierarchy of ISHs, the highest levels transcending our usual bounds and approaching spiritual entities described only in religion. To Watkins and Braun, ISHs more closely resemble all-knowing ego states with their own limitations and personality quirks. Watkins (1980) points out that what they have in knowledge they may lack in power for action or there would be no further problem. He discusses this in some depth as follows:

> The ISH which is all-knowing, hence has within a common cathexis an awareness of the contents of all (or many) ego states, could not possibly be able to extend controlling behaviors or true experiential perception over all. Because if it could these states would not be dissociated but a unity. Efforts to force the "all-

knowing" one to take behavioral and experiential responsibility must fail as long as the need for dissociation exists. The dissociation is maintained, but along a different axis.

If pathological ego states A and B are separated as if beside one another, the ISH could be described as an awareness of A and B experiences and behaviors, but only at an intellectual content level. The split here is not that of one ego state from another *per se*, but between cognitive awareness and power for action. Seeing multiplicity as a complex form of spontaneous hypnosis corresponds to Hilgard's description of the separation in hypnosis between the observing and executive functions of the central executive (Hilgard, 1977).

Like hidden observers, ISHs present a new datum, an unknown. They are now part of the reservoir of data which science seeks to explain, so far without success. One can only speculate on the broader philosophical implications of the hidden observers and ISHs, which I suspect are similar and present in everybody at all times. While one could hypothesize that a hidden observer or ISH could be personified and talked to only in hypnosis and equivalent pathological states, the positioning of both hypnosis and dissociation along a continuum with no measurable boundary between A and Not-A suggests that what occurs within A must also occur beyond, thus pointing to a new dimension of human life worth close study.

To the clinician, the challenge presented by the ISH is whether it can be activated and given power, rectifying the split between the knowledge and power for action which has been described by Watkins. While it might have power for action only when there is no further need for pathological or dysfunctional dissociation, its information content could certainly facilitate that outcome.

6

Treatment of

Dissociative Disorder

The first dilemma posed by dissociative disorder to the clinician is the question of whether it is meaningful and useful for him to perceive alter-personalities and their ego state equivalents within a given patient as having a unique sense of identity of their own. Should he seek out, find and communicate with many different parts of that patient toward the end of helping him integrate these creatively into a Cohesive Self? Or would treating him as a unified whole to begin with prove more efficacious? Since every individual is actually both a whole as well as composed of many parts, like any complex organization, the issue becomes the question of which conceptualization is the more useful.

Familiar with all the Eves and the Sybils, many practitioners assiduously avoid dealing with a dissociating patient as a multiple personality for fear of therapeutic artifact. They raise the issue that an assortment of undesirable outcomes might result from inadvertent hypnotic suggestion, from a patient's desire to please a therapist known to have interest in such phenomena or even from the way language is used when talking about a multiple personality.

This therapeutic approach, it is argued, could for one thing have

111

the effect of actually creating something presumed not only to be non-existent, but also unnecessary and undesirable, i.e., an iatrogenic monster. It is further objected that through such devices as identifying alter-personalities or calling them forth by name, boundaries might be rigidified, reinforcing the very "pathology" we are supposed to be treating, or that such broad use of the multiple personality framework might "foster pathological defenses."

All these considerations boil down to one or two philosophical questions: To what extent, if at all, can people actually create "reality" through their beliefs and expectations? Roberts (1974) argues that this is possible not only with psychic but even physical reality! And to what extent can that reality justifiably be assumed to be bad? Without this covert assumption of the "badness" of multiple personality, arguments against treatment of dissociative disorder as multiple personality would be hollow.

Bearing in mind that either the multiplicity or the unity framework—and often both—might be valid for many patients, the above concerns become a matter of pragmatics. What is most useful? What works? The other side of the coin is shown by the empirical data of many patients who were successfully treated only after a diagnosis of multiple personality was made and corresponding treatment appropriately instituted.

I will deal in turn with the concerns which have been raised. There can be little doubt that a multiple personality syndrome can be created or at least surface through a therapeutic maneuver. This is possible through direct suggestion with over half of highly hypnotizable subjects. Moreover, the work of Harriman (1943) shows spontaneous emergence of alter-personalities in normal subjects in response to a simple hypnotic negation of self. But is it not more likely that the alter-personality was already there? Unless we believe in creation from nothing, the alter-personality, though not a multiple personality syndrome as defined earlier, must already have been present in at least latent form even in Harriman's normal subjects. However, for a psychiatric diagnosis of multiple personality to hold water, the syndrome itself must have been present prior to hypnotic or therapeutic intervention. This is why most clinicians who treat these disorders require documentation from ancillary sources as a criterion of definitive diagnosis.

In more cases than we are generally aware of, this diagnosis is all that can make sense of continuing history of chaotic seeming contradictions.

Is the syndrome unnecessary? Probably and hopefully so, or we would not be seeing the patient in therapy. Yet if it is there, it is there to be dealt with. And it is hardly unnecessary to the patient himself, who would not otherwise have created it.

And is the multiple personality syndrome necessarily bad? This, more than any other assumption I am dealing with, must be called into question. A single, gigantic, undifferentiated oneness cannot necessarily be considered a healthier condition than a complex cooperative whole comprised of many functioning subparts, like orchestra members, their power for action enhanced by division of labor.

I often wonder whether a viable treatment modality for borderlines whose splitting is too chaotic to qualify as multiples might not actually be to purposefully create a multiple personality syndrome, organizing collections of relatively compatible behaviors and experiences into "entities" which then can be further integrated. Though not yet tested, this could be a step toward a higher organization which, though still inadequate, might give us a handle to grasp, permitting treatment modalities far more time- and cost-efficient than the conventional type of psychoanalysis generally accepted so far as the only definitive treatment for borderlines in today's armamentarium.

If Braun's super-multiples are identical to patients I simply term borderline, this not only negates the apparent contradiction between his and my findings referred to earlier, but also dovetails this hypothesized treatment modality with that which Braun already uses (1979, 1980). Start with 40 and gradually integrate the set to 10, then four, then two — and at last a whole person emerges in the usual sense of the term.

To reemphasize the therapeutic issue, the task is not to determine whether or not dissociating is "bad," but to change dysfunctional into useful dissociating, so that a symptom becomes a skill. Many treatment dilemmas emerge. Present in any psychotherapy context, they are set forth in relief in the treatment of multiple personalities and their equivalents. As discussed later in this chapter, the way these dilemmas are dealt with in the multiplicity context should have mental health ramifications far beyond the diagnostic category of major dissociative disorder *per se*. Multiple personality, a therapeutic challenge in itself, is also seen as a paradigm to be extended widely in directions unique to each practicing therapist, as well as to his or her clients.

While treatment issues are manifold and complex, the overriding theme is to avoid the "illness" or "psychopathology" model with its powerfully indelible covert stigma of negative value judgment, defect or not-OKness. In defining the symptom instead as a skill not being used so effectively as one would like — a formulation equally true and more compatible with the patient's sense of pride — dissociation can be seen as an aspect of the hypnotic process. With capacity for autohypnosis acknowledged by many as one of humankind's greatest assets, a logical treatment rationale then emerges. It involves invoking voluntary executive control to convert symptom to skill; basic faith and adequate information exchange are essential to the process.

I will return to prevailing dilemmas in a later discussion, after a survey of pertinent principles in the treatment of dissociative disorder.

TREATMENT PRINCIPLES

Validation and Protection

High therapeutic priority is given to achieving rapport at as many levels as reasonably possible. The primary vehicle for this is what I refer to as *validation* or the process of communication whereby another individual or part-self feels that he is seen, heard and taken seriously.

Yet, supervening this is the even higher priority of life preservation. More often than not a multiple personality will first come to psychiatric attention in such a crisis that there is significant risk of imminent harm to himself or others. Since no amount of validation or rapport can assist a patient who is either dead or sentenced to life imprisonment, *protection* must take priority over validation in real life crises. Actually, even when forcefully and strenuously opposed, protection is usually interpreted correctly as validation by some important part-self that had up to that point not been given adequate attention. Since validation and protection go hand in hand, I will treat them as one.

For the same reasons which led to the splitting and disowning in the first place, awareness of and contact with a formerly hidden alter-personality may be a terrifying if not overwhelming experience. Validation is hence not without some inherent risks. Alcohol binges, suicide attempts, and reckless behavior putting both self and others at risk are not uncommon responses, often in frightful proportions. Rarely, an activated alter-personaliy may even be actively homicidal.

As I become skilled in indirect validation of alter-personalities and increasingly comfortable with a more gradual approach compatible with outpatient treatment (which sometimes has more rapid results), I find regressive behavior less intense. When it is present and severe, however, protection must be provided by any available means, which can include involuntary commitment, seclusion, restraints and/or doses of medication ordinarily considered extreme.

Distinctly contraindicated are any "I'm only trying to help you" games. What is necessary is a firm, caring statement that protection is and will continue to be provided by whatever means necessary, making priorities clear.

Life preservation, as well as inability to care for one's own basic needs, may call for inpatient hospital treatment. I often prefer to undertake definitive diagnosis and treatment in a hospital setting so that forceful protection can be rapidly assured if needed.

The first order of business therapeutically is validation of not only the patient's primary personality—i.e., his usual personality state, often bewildered, amnesic and chronically depressed—but also his alter-personalities. This presents some logistic problems, for often the part-selves are so discordant that what will satisfy one will antagonize another. A cardinal rule is to *be aware that others are listening in*—alter-personalities, ego states, ISHs, etc. Any "reassurance" that makes an enemy of a significant alter-personality will sabotage treatment at the onset.

Hiding behind the popular rationalization that the "narcissistic transference" is too severe for a patient to evaluate a therapist's behavior accurately is dangerously fallacious, neglecting convincing data on the presence of excellent ISHs and hidden observers even in the most disturbed of borderlines. The therapist's attitude should in many ways be like that of a careful CIA agent in the field, saying only what he is willing for any potential listener to hear.

Circumstances are similar to those in skilled family therapy, another setting in which making an enemy of any significant component member might render the entire treatment ineffectual. The Watkins (1979b) even define their "ego state therapy" modality as the use of group and family therapy techniques to deal with the "family of Self" comprising a single human individual. Gently extending this principle to cover almost the whole of psychotherapy, Watkins says (1979),

> With any patient I assume that in a sense there are at least two "personalities." One wants to get well or he would not be here in my office. The other does not want to get well or he would already be well.

The wrong kind of reassurance to the first of these two personalities could make an enemy of the second, sabotaging treatment. Perhaps this is the primary etiology of resistance. If so, much resistance may be unnecessary.

An elegant way to indirectly validate a patient's multiple levels is paradoxical permission or positive reframing. Watzlawick, Weakland and Fisch (1974) indicate that the best way to get a resistant patient to move in psychotherapy may be by the paradoxical caution to "go slow." This is not just paradox, but also a literal, valid permission; the therapist cautions the patient to move slowly, considering the disadvantage of change and the exceptional assets of current skills (symptoms) before even contemplating the possibility of change.

The old adage, "When in doubt, go slow," is good advice. The patient should refuse to make major personal changes without adequate information. Besides being uncommon sense, this may be a first step toward making a potent ally of a powerful part-self which might otherwise resist or even undermine treatment. Positive reframing — turning attention to the positive functions of what the patient himself usually considers negative — has the double advantage of making friends of powerful secondary personalities and of allaying anxiety in the primary. A good start.

Information

Almost routinely, dissociating patients are intellectually brilliant, having a nearly insatiable curiosity for understanding, as well as a desire to feel and function better. They are bright, curious — and baffled. If it were possible to describe a multiple by a single word, that word would be "confused." "I just don't know what the heck is going on. Nothing makes any sense," etc. Providing such simple information as has been discussed in this book often has what seems like miraculous results in the "pure psychotherapy" frame. Information that clarifies while preserving the patient's OK sense of pride has the triple advantages of utilizing his intellectual ability and curiosity as an asset; helping him make sense of his problem, thereby giving and increasing motivation; and putting him more in charge of his own therapy—all most desirable goals.

I am increasingly impressed and often astounded by the dramatic turning points in therapy developing around a simple informational lecture, to the point that I suggest it become a necessary part of standard treatment. Berne (1961) founded transactional analysis partly on the premise that simple language, shared between patient and therapist in easy lay terms that are still professionally precise, has this very type of value. When the therapist enhances rather than sacrifices the patient's sense of OKness, the patient becomes a more active collaborator in his own therapy. Properly conveyed, an informational discussion of dissociation emphasizing the dimensions of a dysfunctional versus useful ability, as opposed to a diagnosis of psychopathology, may have a significant impact on the course of therapy. I am hopeful this may be a major way out of the reparenting equivalents still resorted to by so many practitioners in this field.

Internal Self-Helpers

Allison's (1974) discovery of the internal self-helper (ISH) is a major event and milestone in understanding and dealing with dissociation. There is increasing agreement that the ISH is similar to Hilgard's hidden observer, most clinicians now believing that it goes beyond the paradigm of objective data-processing he described, with a potentially infinite number of ISHs, each having personality characteristics of its own. Watkins and Watkins (1980) point out that the ISH properly equates only with that hidden observer capable of being a true helper, as opposed to other hidden observers serving the sole purpose of passive observation, though surely the value of pure information-gathering is not to be discounted.

Therapeutically, the ISH should be a great asset in treatment of a multiple. Early accessing of the ISH can clarify the therapist's proper strategy, if nothing more — no mean feat in the case of patients who uniformly tax the resources of the most brilliant and experienced clinicians. Watkins comments that what the ISH has in knowledge it may lack in power for whatever reason — or else the problem would have already been solved. Understanding is dissociated from power for action. When this is corrected, the ISH can become an even more potent therapist than the practitioner himself, a knowledgeable, effective self-therapist. Perhaps this is a good end point of formal psychotherapy — seeking not "cure," whatever that may mean, but ability of the patient to take charge of his own continuing growth, extending throughout a long and productive life.

Another summary maxim: When in difficulty, step out of the therapeutic frame and simply ask the patient, or his ISH, his beliefs about the problem and the best course of action. Generally, productive work rapidly resumes.

Allison distinguished ISHs most carefully from "pathological" alter-personalities in having 1) no identifiable time and purpose of origin; 2) having no defensive function; 3) being all-knowing; 4) being incapable of transference and therefore able to point out the therapist's mistakes, a sobering thought; and 5) perhaps even extending in some hierarchical fashion with psychological "entities" beyond usual physical boundaries.

This merges closely with expansive alternative viewpoints about reality posed by such investigators as Roberts (1972), going far beyond scientific testing but to be ignored only at risk — if only the risk of sacrificed potency. The issues raised by Roberts (1974) as a person are inescapable, since she writes provocative books on many topics in entirely different personality states, using these (even with partial to total amnesia) to the highest productive ends. While she is no more satisfied than I with the number of typically spiritualistic interpretations of her work, much information is there in print to be examined by anybody willing to risk expanding his outlook on the nature of life and of man.

I suspect that further insight from continuing research and clinical work with hidden observers and internal self-helpers will transform our conception of humanness in ways we can only speculate upon at present. For now, it is best to treat each case as a new datum, keeping all senses sharp with a willingness to apply whatever we observe to the best therapeutic end. The result will be both greater flexibility as therapists and accumulation of an increasing body of unbiased information for further scientific scrutiny.

General Treatment

Since every therapist has his own individualized way of working and does best by developing and refining his own style, I prefer to outline basic issues at the relative expense of my more specific *modus operandi*. Salient features to be emphasized include 1) general ego building, including critical basic care of body and mind; 2) lowering of amnesic barriers, to foster the intrapsychic flow of information required for coherent cooperative functions; and 3) taking charge, from the point of view of a competent overall executive or conductor, so that what was once a symptom becomes a skill.

Basic body care includes proper nutrition, exercise, rest and maintenance of physiological needs. Few individuals deny that they function better when in optimal physical health and this seems especially true with psychiatric patients. With major dissociative disorder, where the internal fragmentation and warfare may be perceived as a terrifying threat even to survival, the patient cannot afford to sacrifice any of the strength afforded by basic health. If the patient is threatened by chronic medical ailments, he should be under close professional supervision and treatment, the doctor working in collaboration with the therapist.

People differ in opinion as to proper care of the mind. As indicated above, multiple personalities are generally brilliant, with an insatiable curiosity about themselves and life issues. Optimal *intellectual stimulation* can then help refine and develop that curiosity which, if well employed, is capable of becoming one of the patient's greatest assets for treatment, besides helping him with the many challenges he will continue to face throughout his lifetime.

I usually suggest reading material bearing upon the patient's problem at a high intellectual level, requesting his feedback not only as patient but also as critic. Besides facilitating the build-up of information, this provides potent indirect validation of his ability to carry on autonomously outside the therapeutic situation. Self-assessment questionnaires are also potent devices for focusing the patient's intellectual skill and bringing it to bear upon his problems. A variant that sometimes validates stubbornly resistant part-selves is an assignment to list the *dis*advantages of positive change. Underlying the accessing of his intellectual skills is the "go slow" permission.

THERAPEUTIC HYPNOSIS AND ITS EQUIVALENTS

Therapeutic hypnosis has been inextricably associated with diagnosis and treatment of dissociative disorder as long as the latter has been recognized, as has been described by Braun (1980). I define therapeutic hypnosis in a somewhat different way than I have defined hypnosis in the scientific context of Chapter 2, but one which is entirely compatible with that. In the broadest sense, which includes what I term "hypnotic equivalents," I use the definition of Erickson (Beahrs, 1971) that hypnosis is simply *"communication with the unconscious."* Since what is "unconscious" is relative, all parts having a simultaneous conscious experience of their own, I would rephrase this definition as communication with aspects of the patient or subject which are normally beyond control or awareness of the person's executive or conductor. By *formal* hypnosis, I refer to the process where a subject begins in a "non-hypnotic" state, and by means of a formal series of variably ritualized and variably individualized communications, goes through a transition phase or induction, resulting in a distinctly different state of mind called "trance." Formal hypnosis shares with hypnotic equivalents the very criteria by which I defined hypnosis in Chapter 2: increased spontaneity or involuntary quality of movements and experiences, fluidity of perception, and flexibility and increasingly regressed modes of cognition.

As the essence of psychotherapy within the multiplicity model is communicating with and enhancing communication among all parts of an individual, therapeutic hypnosis or its equivalents pervades the entire process, and most of the techniques described in this book fit into this rubric. Everything which can be done by formal hypnosis I believe can be done equally well with informal hypnosis and hypnotic equivalents; the more I become skilled at the latter the less I use the former. As I have elsewhere claimed (Beahrs, 1982), the hypnotic equivalent of communicating at the same time with many otherwise "hidden" parts of self is what gave Milton Erickson's psychotherapeutic technique such a seemingly bizarre quality, as well as its decisive effectiveness.

Formal hypnosis and its equivalents are used in basically two ways in the treatment of dissociative disorder. The first is general treatment, and can be applied to almost any individual with any type of problem with likelihood that it will be of value. This is simply to enhance the person's own skill at autohypnosis, helping him to be able to experience the wide gamut of hypnotic phenomena under voluntary control so that what had either been a symptom or at least an untapped potential now becomes a skill of the highest order. For a "good" hypnotic subject, formal hypnosis and increased experience with the hypnotic phenomenon itself have this desirable outcome even as an artifact.

The second use of hypnosis and its equivalents, specifically tailored to dissociative disorder, is the use of this modality to call forth or elicit alter-personalities or part-selves which otherwise are rarely seen except when out of control, and to access them in a controlled setting. This is considered the treatment of choice by most investigators in this field.

Multiple personalities have proven nearly universally to be good hypnotic subjects, so the induction of a deep hypnotic trance by standard inductions has never proven to be of great difficulty. Prior to hypnosis I have always asked the primary patient for permission to access and talk to a part or parts that might be hidden. Once the patient is in a trance, I ask to speak to the usually hidden alter-personality; when I make contact with that part, I attempt to get to know him almost the same way I would get to know any new individual. I give suggestions for how an alter-personality can be accessed, as well as for how it can be deaccessed, and generally ask and obtain permission from the alter-personality as well as the primary personality for relief of the amnesic barriers. When either part is reluctant to let go of the amnesic barrier, it has always been willing to accept a suggestion that "when ready" the intrapsychic information flow will increase, and this has usually occurred within no more than a week or two.

But awareness of a demonic alter-personality is often terrifying to a scared primary, who is chronically depressed and experiences only a very limited ability at coping. To suddenly have a hypermanic, apparently powerful, and grandiose competitor banging at the door of the self is terrifying, to say the least, especially when the primary self fears, not without reason, that the secondary might get the whole personality into great difficulties by his or her aberrant behavior.

While formal hypnosis has the obvious advantages of rapidly improving intrapsychic information exchange and the potential for learning voluntary control, there is a difficulty which has been so persistent and vexing that I have increasingly avoided the modality of formal hypnosis. Since awareness of the full extent of what is dissociated is so terrifying, the primary may become very resistant to further psychotherapy and to hypnosis in particular. Interestingly, it is the *primary* ("conscious" in the usual sense) that becomes resistant, not the secondary part or "demon" which had been hidden. If the initial therapeutic transactions are well done, the demon is often all too eager to become a cooperative part, and it is the patient in his usual self role who becomes resistant.

In one case I had done some decisive work with a patient and her secondary personality, which led to a full information exchange and peaceful coexistence almost equivalent to a fusion. A year later, under stress, she decompensated and again split and started suppressing her demon, which resumed acting out and sabotaging the patient's life. This time, when I saw her and again wanted to talk with her secondary personality, she openly resisted. "Why are you showing so much interest in *her* (alter-personality)? Don't *I* have any rights? Do I not matter to you? Was it not I who saw you first? All I hear is her, her, her." Here I was in a true therapeutic triangle — a triangle between two part-selves who were competing for affection just as if they were separate females.

Narcissistic pride as a determinant in healthy human living has only recently been given attention, and usually only in a negative vein. Yet it is a fact of life to be dealt with. I think much of Milton Erickson's genius lay in recognizing the importance of this pride, and communicating with secondary parts of a personality *indirectly* so that it would not be threatened. It was an intuitive awareness on Erickson's part that resistance would come from the *conscious* or the primary *self*, when this pride was threatened, much more than from the unconscious who would all too willingly cooperate if given a chance.

Alter-personalities can be accessed in a variety of direct and indirect ways. The most direct, but also much like a bull in a china shop, is the method of formal hypnosis and direct hypnotic suggestion, with the attendant difficulties just described. More elegant techniques can follow from the simple awareness of the fact that there are multiple consciousnesses listening in on what we are saying, whether we are directing our words to them or not; how these are reacting can often be presumed by observation of nonverbal responses to our communication. Spontaneous body movements which are incongruent with the patient's words are communication from a patient at a different level, well known to psychotherapists of all disciplines. When we note a person's head shaking no, we might simply ask the patient what his head is saying. Nervous laughter followed by noticeable relaxation and deep breaths indicates that an important part of the patient's personality knows he is being taken seriously and is relaxing the pressure and expressing his appreciation. Often that part will express himself fully at that point, without the primary having been forced out of the way by a hypnotic bludgeon. Finger signals as a way of communicating with the unconscious (LeCron, 1964) are another method par excellence of knowing when a secondary part-self is accessible. I am increasingly impressed with how often spontaneous finger signals with their own idiosyncratic meaning are present even in individuals without any prior hypnotic or therapeutic experience.

Learning the meaning of idiosyncratic body movements is a potent way of enhancing intrapsychic information exchange and communication, without the therapeutic bludgeon of formal hypnosis. Acting on a therapeutic hunch is sometimes of value. "If I were in your position, I would probably want to . . ." may elicit a strong validating reaction from an alter-personality who is there and indeed experiencing things as hypothesized.

Two-chair techniques, as employed by Gestaltists, are a potent method of separating parts in conflict, and accessing and validating the needs of both. I described these as a variant of hypnotic technique (Beahrs & Humiston, 1974), and find that the same principle can be employed effectively without having to use two different physical chairs. Projecting oneself into dream elements, either with or without the two-chair technique, can be a powerful way of accessing whatever was represented by said dream element, and is remarkably easy to do. If one aspect of a personality is rigidly holding on to its control, the therapist mimicking that part which is in control might elicit a response from the opposite polarity in cases where the two-chair work was ineffective.

While I have talked somewhat disparagingly of formal hypnosis as like a "bludgeon," I believe that it has its place and that it is effective if the needs of all parts of the personality are taken into account. Encouraging increased attentiveness to nonverbal signals, whether they be head movements or finger movements or spontaneous visual images, invariably results in hypnotic trance. The attitude of expectancy towards spontaneous communication both enhances the latter and sets aside the conscious controlling functions, which is almost the definition of what hypnosis itself is. Hence, it is not either/or — we can have the best of both worlds.

Enhancing a patient's *hypnotic experience* in a controlled setting is another ego-building therapeutic tool. Erickson (Beahrs, 1971) long maintained that the subject's experiencing a wide range of hypnotic behavior, even when it was not specifically tailored to his own problems, led to desirable therapeutic change and growth that could seem to just happen. This is especially true for those individuals whose presumed pathology could be looked upon as autohypnosis not optimally used, a basic premise of this inquiry. Learning to use autohypnosis as a skill in a variety of neutral areas cannot help spilling over into the emotionally charged areas of the subject's life, which he can then take under his umbrella at his own leisure even without therapeutic assistance. When direct therapeutic intervention is required, as in first accessing and talking with persecutory part-selves, hypnotic ability is also a prime asset. Hypnosis is the most reliable way known to date for calling forth a hidden alter-personality in a way that enhances control, while potentially validating the needs of all discordant part-selves comprising the treatment situation.

Lowering amnesic barriers is a *sine qua non* for effective treatment of a dissociating patient. The formerly dissociated part-selves are first viewed as object. While that which had been disowned is often terrifying to the usual self when first faced, re-owning it as part of the self is necessary before the patient can become a cohesive whole in any meaningful sense. A conductor cannot organize his orchestra if he is unaware of what a large section of it is even doing; yet this is the state of affairs maintained by an amnesic barrier. While hypnosis is a potent vehicle for enhancing memory, if amnesic barriers are lifted too suddenly the resulting anxiety may lead unnecessarily to resistance to further work. Still, that lifting may never occur if it is determined solely by when the patient is "ready." Titrating increasing awareness to an optimal rate and level is a skill psychotherapists can learn only through experience.

The conductor has jurisdiction over only what is defined as part of his own specific orchestra, not musical groups outside his. Following release of amnesic barriers, then, the executive must not only see and hear the formerly disowned part-selves, but re-own them as part of his overall Self, as subject instead of object. This is equally true from the perspective of that part-self who must accept that he is an important facet of a greater overall whole, an awareness that need not deprive him of his unique individuality. This often takes time, persistence, patience and skill — on the part of the patient as much as the therapist.

Taking charge, so that what was once a symptom becomes a skill, is the therapeutic end point. In the case of Mrs. R cited earlier, this took barely 20 minutes. When part-selves are rigidly separated from or discordant with one another, it is not so easy. If an overall executive or conductor is not clearly defined, different part-selves will vie with one another for the conductor's baton. There are no rules accepted across the board even by experienced therapists as to who should take the baton. The primary personality, "original" personality, most healthy secondary personality, and an ISH have all been declared as candidates, no rule of procedure having withstood all the tests.

Each case must be decided on its own merits. The therapist can only be a potent facilitator or internal diplomat, the decision necessarily having to be made by the collective of part-selves comprising the patient's whole personality. What is required is that there be some persistent organizing force or central executive, however set up and maintained in office, and that he as well as his constituents know who is in charge and who is responsible for what. Only then can the individual function harmoniously like an orchestra, a cohesive whole comprised of parts that take joy in their own individuality, all doing what they do best.

PERSECUTOR ALTER-PERSONALITIES

Dissociating patients who come to psychiatric attention generally have one or more part-selves that can be defined by the majority of their behaviors as "persecutor personalities," whose behavior adversely affects the overall Self and perhaps other individuals as well. The primary or usual self struggles to disown the other part(s), by which it believes itself to be victimized, by maintaining the amnesic barrier. The secondary personality is only too pleased to have this protection behind which to hide, so the amnesic barrier is most likely the responsibility of both parts, a "collusion between part-selves" or responsibility of the entire Self.

Yet in the clinical syndrome, the impasse is beyond voluntary control of any part-self alone. Since they are not in sufficient communication to remedy this, we have indeed a true symptom. At different levels, the patient is either responsible or not responsible for this position, with implications that are complex both legally and therapeutically. How do we deal with persecutors? I will outline my own working principles here and elaborate upon them more fully in the following chapter with clinical case material.

Making Friends of Demons

What I call simply a "demon" is close to what Sullivan (1953) terms the not-me, Lowen (1967) calls demons and monsters, and Berne (1972) terms a Child-demon as opposed to Parent-demon. Far and away the most common type of persecutory alter-personality, it is at the same time one of the most flamboyant and terrifying to most people, as well as, fortunately, the most benign and accessible. This is not to say that demons don't do enough evil deeds to justify their name; many of history's greatest atrocities are probably their responsibility. What I am emphasizing is the critical necessity of being precise and accurate about where value judgments are appropriate. Value judgments, in my (as well as most therapists') opinion, are appropriate to behaviors only — definitely not to the basic being of any individual or even any part. This includes his feelings, all of which comprise a part of basic being. I am conveniently ignoring consideration of those thoughts that may present a gray in-between area. The major concern is to avoid the category error of placing value judgments upon the basic being or the feelings of any part-self. I suspect that some degree of this judgmental category error may be necessary for the maintenance as well as formation of demons as separate alter-personalities or there would be no subjective need to disown any aspect or part of self. Instead, it would be more useful to accept all parts as OK, at the same time as taking voluntary control of all behaviors and responsibility for them. While I believe this simple error of logic plays a major role in the vast majority of psychiatric disorders, nowhere is it exemplified so clearly and unavoidably as in the formation and maintenance of demons as well as in their therapy.

As I use the term, the demon is largely pure life energy. Initially suppressed and disowned out of fear, it then turns back against the self in rage. What we see as a persecutor is merely a normal child response to being the recipient of persecution, that rejection inherent in the original disowning or suppression. This reversal is *the* critical awareness for making friends with a demon, who may then become the patient's greatest asset.

Remembering the "everybody is listening in" rule, a stock reply to a patient's wanting to be "rid of" something about himself — often that which he perceives as a demon (thus the term) — is "Why would you want to 'get rid of' an important part of your own basic being?" The patient may do a double-take and enter into careful thought, while the demon senses a potential ally and relaxes some, allaying some of the anxiety in the primary patient as well. A beneficient circle may already be in the offing. If a patient angrily says "I hate myself!!" I may unobtrusively ask how it feels to *be* hated by one's own self, generally eliciting a response from a secondary part of either sadness, bitterness or rage. In a classic demon, the reply is to disown its sadness and to take sadistic delight in describing his means of torturing his victim, in a way both terrifying and yet likely to arouse vicarious delight in most listeners. Here, as in a great flood, is the patient's life energy, formerly experienced as not-me.

Treatment of anything so important as one's basic life energy is clearly not a matter of "getting rid of," but of accepting it and directing it positively. In dissociative disorder, this involves working with both parts. With the primary, it generally involves dealing with the pathogenic category error, fostering the life-supporting Big P — *Permission to Be* — permission for all parts of the self to exist, which also subtly implies that behaviors can be placed under adequate control.

The first step is to treat the demon respectfully and diplomatically, conveying at least the therapist's permission to exist as a legitimate part and asking what that part would really like to have happen if everything could go his way. Considering that this may be the first time in its life history the demon has ever been treated with respect,

its rapid rapport and malleability may seem remarkable. When the
alienation and trench warfare between part-selves has been more
severe, however, as in the classic multiples, a stronger tack may be required.

In at least 50 percent of classic demons I have worked with, there
has been a transaction with the demon that is almost stereotyped.

> *Demon:* He is so weak and pathetic he might as well be put out
> of his misery. I'm going to help him kill himself so he can get
> some rest.
>
> *Therapist:* You say you live for the sheer joy of living. Where
> will you be then?
>
> *Demon:* Hmmm, that's interesting (dispassionately); I hadn't
> thought of that.

Although he had truly not thought of the obvious, there was no
resistance to hearing and accepting it. After that the demon became a
friend—and quickly. What may be the major transaction can be as
fast as that, right then and there, and often with little if any discom-
fort. This is quite sobering to those therapists who cling to the belief
that only a prolonged working through can achieve meaningful therapeutic change. While no two individuals are alike, it is remarkable
how often some variant of the above seems to happen, even with the
multiple etiologies already discussed.

Another factor to keep in mind with demons is that the demon may
be unwilling to part with his experience of separate identity, perhaps
to avoid experiencing the primary's unnecessary suffering or perhaps
to "protect" the primary from his own "foolishness"—perhaps both. I
believe that therapy works better when this wish is respected, contrary
to those who see fusion as the ultimate ideal. I can find nothing unhealthy in an individual with two relatively separate but cooperative
subparts.

The primary self welcomes the infusion of long-lost life energy that
the erstwhile demon provides. The demon welcomes the protection
the primary's structure and executive control provide, for a typical
demon wants nothing of responsibility, yet knows and appreciates that
behavior control is to everyone's interest. This is simply natural division
of labor at its best. Also, it is not unlike the separation of ego states described by transactional analysts as the normal state of affairs.

Resistant Persecutors

Allison (1977) lists as a stage in his treatment paradigm "getting rid of persecutors." This alarms me, as it not only plays into the original pathogenic category error but also is persecutory in itself. I know few things that any organism is more resistant to than dying; any part-self perceiving itself as a whole organism would fight any threat of annihilation with the full force of its life instinct. Steiner (1979) defines a Pig as the primitive Parent in the Child, the purveyor of dangerous "Don't be" messages, always wrong and bad. Such a negative "always" position would feed any paradigm suggesting that we abolish something. If this "something" has an experience of its own, it may behave with the desperation of a cornered animal when threatened, this behavior seeming so persecutory to the usual self and others as to reinforce the belief that it should be done away with.

I do not accept that any part-self is so bad in its basic being that it should be exterminated and doubt that such riddance is even possible short of biological death. Even if it were, whether this would be desirable is open to question. This raises another philosophical issue that must be faced in working with multiple personalities, at a level beyond psychiatry in general. This is the question of what we mean by death—of either a whole organism or any part experiencing itself as such. This must be discussed with a resistant part-self from the perspective of that part's subjective experience, not the patient's or therapist's overall world view. I will return to this topic when discussing fusion.

One particularly resistant persecutor is described in greater depth in the following chapter, discussed as a tyrant. While this is close to a personification of Steiner's Pig, I prefer the words *tyrant* or *bully* as more descriptive and somewhat less judgmental. The significant thing here is that what initially seemed to patient and therapist alike devoid of any redeeming value whatsoever was subsequently revealed to carry the greatest part of this patient's life energy. That energy had seemed missing because it was associated with a Child ego state so terrified of annihilation as to keep hidden for self-protection. The tyrannical behavior itself was an indirect expression of this primal fear and a primitive attempt to provide that protection.

From the point of view of such an ego state, any attempt to abolish or even neutralize him—a far better term than "get rid of"—could have been perceived as a threat to survival. Only when feeling sufficiently safe could this aspect of the tyrant, a personality within a personality, come out. Treatment was then to provide protection by all means possible, including forceful means, which reassured that scared Child at his own level that he was safe.

When a persecutor is overly rigid and tyrannical, especially if the patient's life energy is not visible elsewhere, I am inclined to view him much as I would a tyrant or bully in the outside world—as a scared child who, because of his vulnerability, will not own up to his fear, choosing instead to bully those he can push around. Protecting the tyrant or bully may ultimately prove far more workable than self-defeating attempts to get rid of him. Feeling safe will enable a part-self as well as whole organism to let go of destructive behavior that was harmful to him as well as others. Fromm (1973) and Roberts (1974) both cite destructiveness as coming from a position of power*less*ness. It is precisely the result of this which a therapist, as well as a patient, may perceive as something so bad that it should be exterminated. I hope this awareness will lead to more desirable and productive alternatives.

In actual fact not all alter-personalities may be workable, as much as I would like to believe otherwise. While Allison acknowledges that making allies of persecutors is his first preference, he is skeptical about how often this is possible. Just as persecutory behavior in and between human societies can sometimes be dealt with only by counterforce, even with the same undesirable considerations as apply to within, so may be the case with some part-selves. This may be most true with respect to a long-hidden avenger which does not even emerge until its smouldering rage blows beyond its chains, with a major criminal offense the result.

When a therapist does encounter what appears to be such a negative part, the word "neutralize" should come to mind before "getting rid of." Any possibility of this part's finding a useful role in the family of Self should be sought, and our minds kept open to that eventuality, even when everybody may have given up hope. An experienced therapist will always do what he can to maximize this possibility.

TREATMENT DILEMMAS

Of the many dilemmas these paradoxical dissociative disorders raise for the clinician, the first is deciding whether or not to work within a multiplicity framework to begin with. As discussed at the beginning of this chapter, this may often prove fruitful and for many patients open doors formerly slammed shut. For others, an alternative model such as the many currently in vogue may work better. Many therapists prefer to avoid dealing with even a full-blown multiple personality as such, not only because of fear of the unknown, but also because of concern that the very language employed could either rigidify the boundaries we are supposed to loosening or foster pathological defenses.

Fear of rigidifying boundaries through artifact is a legitimate concern, for simply using language that implies something like rigid boundaries between subparts may often lead to the behavior so implied. Deliberate use of this aspect of language is, in fact, common practice among hypnotherapists. Overly rigid boundaries are generally more of a problem than of any value, however, being Watkins' major criterion for differentiating multiple personality syndromes from the less severe ego state disorders. We are thus in a bind. If we cannot use language in a way that corresponds closely to observable behavior and reportable subjective experience, information exchange and resultant power for action are needlessly abrogated. Yet using language that is sufficiently descriptive may actually reinforce the undesirable rigidities which constitute much of what is being described.

As with many therapeutic problems, I have found no satisfactory alternative to simply discussing the matter factually and impassively with the patient, inviting his thoughts and feedback. Fortunately, this simple information exchange has so far been all that is needed, for rare is the patient who really likes his rigid boundaries between subparts, and equally rare one who does not want to discuss his feelings and behaviors in a simple language shared with the therapist. The simple awareness engendered by the very act of the therapist's sharing his bind and his goals may render the potential problem neutralized.

Fostering pathological defenses is another concern often raised concerning use of the multiplicity concept. There is little question that dissociation in multiples is a defense, using that term literally as a way of coping with real or imagined danger in order to provide protection and reduce anxiety. That the defense is pathological seems equally clear or the patient would not be a patient.

But is the optimal goal abandonment of those defenses, letting go or getting rid of them? Or is it rather their improvement, in the interest of providing better protection, the essence of defense? The problem is not the presence of defenses but the failure of those that are simply not working. How much better it sounds and feels to a patient to perceive himself not as sick or pathological with its accompanying negative value judgment, but as having a potentially valuable skill or coping mechanism he is not yet using effectively. However pathological his behavior may be in a literal sense, he is going to resist with all his might the implied not-OKness inherent in any pathology or "defect" model. Here that deified term "resistance" enters the picture.

How much of this resistance is necessary is open to question. The patient's problems can be interpreted with equal validity as a skill that is simply not at this point effectual. So defined, a patient's motivation can increase dramatically, supported by his enhanced narcissistic pride, instead of being pitted against his narcissistic shame and the resistance this arouses. This is true to a degree of most neurotic symptomatology, but how much more so of dissociative disorder, which is basically, after all, just hypnotic ability not fully under executive control.

Capacity for autohypnosis is indeed one of mankind's greatest assets, as clearly stated by Le Cron (1964). When dissociating is placed under voluntary executive control, not only is it no longer a symptom, but it becomes a skill of the highest order.

MORAL CHOICE

Allison's most significant challenge to the mental health profession (1977) is that we need to stop avoiding the issue of good and evil. Especially in multiple personalities, what is needed for resolution is that the patient make clear-cut moral choices. Allison claims that one of the major etiological factors in multiple personality is the person's straddling the fence morally and separating the parts in conflict instead of resolving the conflict. He considers it imperative that all multiple personalities and their equivalents make a moral choice of existential proportions between good and evil.

While I decry artificially separating good and evil as if they were two separate godlike forces — and am aware that such a category error, in attempting to abolish evil, may consequently lead to it, as witness our great wars — Allison's contention about the importance of moral choice needs to be heard by all therapists loud and clear.

Like many therapists, Erickson is sometimes quoted as saying that "there is no place for theology in mental health." I fear that this misses a vital point. There may be little or no place for rigid, doctrinaire beliefs, a negative aspect of many theologies, in that flexible and adaptive state we call mental health. But what about integrity, the foundation upon which Erickson's own masterful methodologies were built? Without that underlying integrity, all the skill in the world would be like a house without a foundation, a point which may be lost on many pop therapists whose "flow with it" type of ethics is, fortunately, now on the downswing.

Flexibility without integrity is like a house without a foundation or a tree without roots. Integrity without flexibility, on the other hand, quickly becomes a rigidity, which itself can predispose to dysfunctional splitting.

Perhaps the necessary moral choice is to take some stand or life position which defines one's identity, including one's values. One can then become sufficiently rooted in the foundation of one's integrity that the resultant security makes it easier to own up to aspects of oneself perceived as evil, redirecting their energy in desirable directions (good behaviors) as opposed to harmful ones. The relevance of theology to mental health rests not in rigid belief systems but in a faith in the overall OKness of all that is which Lowen (1972), Roberts (1978) and I all see as not only the antithesis of depression, but also the essence of healthy living. Nowhere in our profession is this faith put to a more difficult test than in dealing with those severely dissociated patients whose subparts can challenge virtually everything we have been brought up to believe in.

FUSION OR PEACEFUL COEXISTENCE?

Clinicians working with multiples are sharply divided as to their assessment of the desired end result of treatment. Allison (1979) and Braun (1979) are today's most active proponents of fusion or complete integration of all of the formerly discordant part-selves into a single overall Self, considered necessary before we can meaningfully talk of anything like "cure." Erickson (1976) questions whether this is possible or even desirable and cites Eve's autobiography (Sizemore, 1977) as evidence of successful treatment where alter-personalities neither died nor were swallowed up by the whole Self but cooperated with one another and treated each other with respect. Watkins (1979) makes it clear that fusion as clinically defined is a possible, though not necessarily the most desirable, goal.

"Fused" individuals will not stay fused, for one thing, under conditions meriting further dissociating. Furthermore, if or when fusion does occur, we cannot rationalize away the fact that alter-personalities do die, in exactly the sense in which currently alive human beings look upon death. Death does not mean any loss of spiritual-material substance, but a dissolution of one's experience of an individual self as an entity separate from other entities in time or place. Since a true alter-personality experiences himself as a separate self, he will fight that dissolution with the full force of the self-preservation instinct common to all life. Pragmatically, therefore, cooperation of all parts is more feasible without placing upon them demands they would perceive as unreasonable and non-negotiable. Further, the data of hypnosis show that co-consciousness is the rule rather than the exception. How can we then consider a multiple unhealthy if his part-selves communicate and cooperate with each other under the benign leadership of an executive, like the conductor of the orchestra?

At another level, no part-self actually dies; rather it remains as a latent ego state, a normal part of the personality which may even have its own subjective experience but does not ever "come out" for public view. Watkins' discovery in healthy individuals of potentially infinite latent ego states or hidden observers, which may even have their own unique subjective experiences, raises philosophical issues about the nature of cohesive Self and selves, and their relationship to the universe at large, which are mind-boggling and only beginning to be explored.

For practical reasons, I personally prefer to set the most modest goals that are consonant with healthy living, placing me more in the Erickson and Watkins camp regarding the fusion issue. Particularly interesting is my observation that, when all parts are functioning cooperatively and their right to existence assured, the primary and secondary personalities often become so similar in content and goals as to render separation of little meaning. Or alter-personalities may cease to come out for whatever reason, while retaining the potential. Possibly fusion, behaviorally, is more a by-product than a goal in successful treatment.

Watkins loves social analogies, as do I. His comparison of the splitting of America into Union and Confederacy is a classic example of a "national multiple personality syndrome." With fusion achieved by force, the secondary personality truly died in the usual sense of the term, but not without terrible cost, as well-known to all Americans. A healthy America, as a union of relatively autonomous states, is likened to cooperatively functioning ego states. East and West Germany are more like alter-personalities, with their poor information exchange, poor intercooperation and excessive rigidity of boundaries. Watkins (1979) mentions any expectations of achieving fusion as comparable to "asking the Arabs and Israelis to join together in One Great Big Beautiful Oneness." How *do* we deal with the Arabs and Israelis, a social paradigm of the most difficult dissociative disorders? First, get them to communicate — the all-powerful *information exchange*. Cooperative interplay is the next goal, not yet achieved.

I liken the history of Europe to a gigantic multiple personality. During the Middle Ages, the extreme multiplicity of small feudal fiefdoms was more like a borderline syndrome or those multiples whom Braun describes as having more than 30 identifiable alter-personalities. In the past few centuries, those mutually compatible fiefdoms have coalesced or "fused" into greater part-selves or countries. Yet, their identities are much more separate than those of America's states; we could compare this to the difference between multiple personality and ego state problems. The historical course is parallel to that of many neurotic individuals, with long periods of relative health and cooperation punctuated by crises of the most catastrophic proportions.

Great wars are not unlike a neurotic crisis. Perhaps World War I is a social caricature of the multiple personality syndrome at its very worst — catastrophic, senseless mass destruction with little redeeming value, originating ironically from the nobility of the life instinct, poor information exchange and inability to limit judgments to behaviors and not identities. Is there a better way? Roberts (1976) explicitly cites the parallel between intrapsychic and social politics, and I cannot agree more that learning effective treatment modalities for disturbed patients is one and the same as bettering methods of cooperative international diplomacy.

If we do not seek fusion, we must ask: Who will be in executive control? In his pioneering work on multiplicity, Prince (1906) sought to find the "real" or original personality. He has been followed principally by Allison. But are any existing entities more or less real than others? And is the original personality necessarily the desired one? I, for one, am learning to welcome rather than fear change and have no clear position on this except to strive for whatever works best. The conductor is he who conducts best, considering the unique needs of the overall person.

SUBSTANCE USE

Use of alcohol and medications involves problematic issues. Alcohol, a popular way to bring out a persecutory alter-personality, lessens control, unlike hypnosis. When this is a problem with dissociators, the Alcoholics Anonymous stricture against any alcohol may be the best safeguard. In those alcoholics where dissociation is the primary etiology, cure may subsequently lead to a resumed capacity for social drinking, as contended by Steiner (1971). There may, however, be some difficult testing along the way.

Medications, by and large, are temporary expedients — one of many tools providing forceful protection in severe crisis. Sleeping medications provide still another dilemma, pertinent here because insomnia and resulting use and abuse of medicine are more the rule than the exception with dissociating patients. English (1977), aptly noting that insomnia may represent a primitive equating of sleep with death, suggests that chemically forcing the suppressed healthy part of an individual into submission with pills might be like symbolic suicide, appropriately fought off by that healthy part with all its might. For these as well as dependency reasons she states that sedatives should under no circumstances be used with such patients.

While good reasoning, this fails to take into account the needs of the primary personality, terrified by not sleeping and needing some succor and comfort that the therapist cannot and should not forever be providing. At this level a pill prescribed by a caring physician is an acceptable breast substitute. As in other similar dilemmas, the best one can do is simply discuss the pros and cons with the patient and reach some compromise. The primary personality gets a degree of chemical comfort. The secondary personality, hearing the discussion and knowing he is being taken seriously, is able to accept the evidence that so far the imagined catastrophe of never waking up has not occurred and relaxes. It seems impossible to beat the potency of simple communication.

REPARENTING OR FAITH?

Few beliefs are more uniformly held among therapists than the assumption that dealing with multiple personalities must be hard work—demanding intense commitment of emotional energy and time on the part of the therapist, often at considerable self-sacrifice. If this is done within the spirit of Freud's pioneering explorations in psychoanalysis, toward the main goal of furthering understanding, it is a most rewarding enterprise. Like Freud's work, it may lead to different ways of looking upon ourselves that can point toward new realms of inquiry yet unknown. However, such intense involvement is inefficient of both time and cost when seen purely as treatment of a disturbed patient.

Freud had always maintained that his psychoanalytic method was primarily a research tool, treatment only for the privileged few who could affort the time and expense. He also believed that, if the masses were ever to be reached by psychotherapy, it would have to be through some form of hypnosis. Had his followers taken heed of these words, we would not have had to wait for the recent resurgence in brief therapy modalities derived from hypnosis.

If brief interventions can achieve results comparable to long-term therapy in many neurotic disorders, I would expect this to be expecially true for those patients best seen as simply abusing spontaneous hypnosis in the first place. This was certainly possible with Mrs. R (see Chapter 3), who was able to render her symptom into a skill in one session. With a multiple personality, where the needs of long-entrenched opposing forces may at first seem irreconcilable, I would hardly expect this to occur in 20 minutes. Yet I hope and believe it can occur far more expeditiously than at present.

The more a psychotherapist, over extended time, acts as if he were and should be a new and better parent, what I call reparenting, the more he may try to take over functions that can truly be performed only by the patient. This detracts from a patient's autonomy, which he needs more of, not less.

Multiple personalities can be especially seductive toward a therapist's parental inclinations. The cry of help from a desperate and confused primary personality can be like seeing an abandoned baby lying in the street. The obstinate and petulant behavior of many a secondary personality may provoke a therapist's critical and punitive behavior out of sheer frustration. Since alter-personalities are often largely child ego states, it is not surprising that they should evoke parental responses. These are even asked for and demanded at one level.

The complementary parental behavior of a therapist does not encourage the child-selves of the patient to grow up, however, as it would a real child. It partially gratifies "needs," which more often than not become insatiable. Especially insidious is the implication that the patient cannot serve these functions for himself — that lack of faith inherent in a "defect" model. This comes across loud and clear and may reinforce the patient's feelings of helplessness, while his outwardly helpless behavior reinforces the therapist's reparenting. A system is thereby maintained.

The major hazard as I see it is a type of "therapeutic" symbiosis in which the narcissistic needs of the therapist are gratified as much as those of the patient, perpetuating the original pathogenic binds, much as described by Calof (1979). If the patient frustrates the therapist's narcissistic pride by continuing in his pathology, as well as by not duly appreciating the therapist's efforts, the therapist may not only become angry, but also erupt into full-blown narcissistic rage. Even with these hazards some patients do grow to a successful outcome and, if it is the best we have, it should be used. That a better way is possible is, however, suggested by several encouraging trends.

The careful study of Erickson's techniques now being undertaken is promising, for much of their effectiveness probably lay in his ability to develop rapport and achieve control simultaneously at many levels, precisely what is needed for the dissociator. The *Change* model of the Palo Alto group (Watzlawick, Weakland and Fisch, 1974) outlines a paradigm for brief therapy involving both the paradoxical permission and positive reframing that I am convinced are necessary. The Watkins' formulation of ego state therapy as resembling diplomacy (1978, 1979b) is equally encouraging.

While I have not yet developed the short-cuts I would like to see, I hope that more emphasis upon three factors will lead to increasingly sound and enduring therapeutic results with less expenditure of time and energy by patient and therapist alike. All these factors put the burden of responsibility on the patient for doing what only he can do anyway and enhance a sense of strength to enable him to carry his burden. First is the all-powerful *information exchange*, helping the patient mobilize his intellectual prowess so that it can become the re-source it should be. Second is *strict definition of the therapist's limits* —protecting the patient as much as the therapist by fostering instead of discouraging autonomy and self-therapy. Most critical is the third factor—*faith*—a trust in the OKness of all that is which embraces the therapist and patient and all of their parts.

Regarding limit-setting, the information shared with the patient is a clear, precise and accurate statement of what the therapist can and cannot do. He can talk, write prescriptions, collect fees, authorize hospitalization, administer psychological tests and assume whatever responsibility for his own personal behavior is defined professionally, legally and ethically. He can literally do nothing to or for the patient that is solely the latter's province. Only the patient can cause a glass of gin to touch his lips and the contents to enter his stomach and blood-stream—and only he can prevent such action. Clear precise definition of who does and causes what can clarify and resolve at the outset many potentially dangerous category errors of the type so nearly universal in dissociators and probably most patients in general.

I am experimenting with setting even more restrictive limits on my availability to multiples and borderlines than to others—a reversal of the usual trend. In view of their triple assets of high intelligence and intellectual curiosity, autohypnotic skill and internal self-helpers, I cannot escape the conviction that there must be a better way than over-involvement of the therapist. I may even emphasize that I can*not* be called upon in any crisis (therefore am not indispensable) and am not always willing to hospitalize when the patient wants or feels he needs it. This also helps protect against the sense of betrayal an indi-vidual may feel when at some point his therapist's own humanness unavoidably crosses his own. (However, whenever there is a risk of homicide or suicide, the patient must be hospitalized.)

Perhaps even more important in decreasing dependence upon a therapist is faith — what I see as the ultimate critical factor, even if the least tangible. Conveying confidence that the basic being of all parts is OK lightens the load of anxiety and enables the patient to mobilize his own resources more fully.

All therapists, being human, retain some residual fear of certain aspects of themselves they dislike, which will carry over to corresponding aspects of their patients. Such hesitancy is communicated to the patient and his part-selves at many levels. This gets tricky if we believe that faith as a working position is essential, a point I will develop in a later chapter. When I fear that my own dynamics and prejudices may get in the way, the best way I have found to proceed is to simply discuss this with the patient in an objective, informational manner, sharing only what is necessary to avoid misinterpretation.

Most often this works. Patients are very forgiving of a therapist who can reveal at least a bit of his own humanness within a setting of professional protection, a delicate balance. If he can own up to gaps in his own sense of OKness when these might convey unintentional negative messages to a patient, the therapist will rarely be criticized for being human. When difficulties do arise from covert negative suggestion, "when in doubt, go slow" may become "when in doubt, sweat it out." This is still part of life when working with disturbed patients, who will test a therapist's limits with the most provocative behavior even while secretly hoping these limits will remain firm.

Wholly contraindicated is hiding behind the transference myth. While transference is an observable phenomenon that can and should be utilized when it occurs, the myth is that it alone is all that is happening. This myth should be dispelled once and for all by recognizing that hidden observers and internal self-helpers, present in all, are perceiving the therapist's behavior accurately in spite of whatever transference one ego state might exhibit. The therapist must accept the unavoidable risk of being seen, knowing that mistakes are inevitable and do not contradict anyone's basic value as a therapist or human being.

Ideally, the therapist's role can become more like that of a catalyst, exactly as the term is used in chemistry. While literally doing none of the patient's changing for him, he facilitates it — and hopefully he is a potent facilitator. To what extent this ideal can be approached awaits further research.

7

Working with

Persecutors

Three clinical cases are presented to help illustrate the dilemmas involved in treating persecutory part-selves as we encounter them in clinical practice. The first is an abstract of a characteristic demon, a personification of a patient's vital life energy which had turned against the overall self after it had been disowned and suppressed. The second is a more complicated case of a resistant persecutor which first presented like a tyrant with little redeeming value. The last case clarifies an aspect of internal parenting already raised by the second case. All raise philosophical as well as psychiatric treatment issues that cannot be avoided if these patients are to get better. I will discuss these as they come up after each case presentation, elaborating upon material in the past two chapters.

CASE 1: AN ENCOUNTER WITH A DEMON

The case of Mr. D presented as an abstract of an unsupervised dialogue between a patient's usual self, experiencing himself as a victim, and a personification of what had formerly been seen only as a symptom or "it." This "demon" might have been manifest as neurotic compulsion, phobia, inhibition or substance abuse — all representing the

141

power in what had been disowned. The case is presented as it might occur in a two-chair dialogue common in Gestalt work, with commentary added to advise the therapist on strategies that can be employed at various points to facilitate positive change and protect against danger. The excerpt begins at the point where the patient first becomes aware that what had been experienced only as a neurotic symptom truly has a life and personality of its own. A 30-year-old professional was seeking treatment for chronic depression and a sense of being overwhelmed by stifling "inhibitions." He was asked to place his inhibitions in an empty chair and talk with them.

Dialogue	Commentary
Victim = V	
Demon = D	
V: Why do you inhibit me and cause me so much misery?	Patient is open to new information ("ready to work").
D: Because I don't like you.	An angry child.
V.: Why don't you like me?	
D: Because you're such a sniveling little piece of shit. (Matter-of-fact manner, firmly.)	Latent ego states often show contempt for the primary executive as "weak."
V: Why do you exist? (With increasing look of fear.)	
D: For the sheer joy of torturing you! (With delight—formerly rigid body armor seems to melt, body movements become economical, flowing and graceful, accompanied by a visible and almost overpowering intensity.)	This is *not* a true multiple personality; changes can be equally dramatic in ego state dilemmas.
V: Where did you come from?	
D: Does it matter? I just simply exist for the sheer joy of existing.	The essence of life.
V: (Desperately.) What can I do?	
D: (With sadistic glee.) Nothing, but I just love your	Only the "demon" uses the term "love." He has rarely been out—

impotent struggling—keep it up!

V: Did I get you from my father?

D: Don't give *him* the credit— it's *me* that deserves it! As I said, I exist merely because I exist—for the sheer joy of existence is in torturing you.

the only power he has is better than none.

Life is its own reason—all that is. Behaviorally, if we ignore verbal content, the "demon" shows by far the most positive life force.

V: (Pleading, intellectualizing.) You are driving me crazy, I can't stand it. I have my re-sponsibilities to do. What if I start hearing voices when I'm at a critical point in my work?

D: (Smacking his lips, as if about to devour a delicious morsel.) Oh—that would be lovely!

V: (Exclaims with angry desper-ation.) You're *pure evil!* Something this rotten has *no right to exist* on the face of this earth!

D: (With apparent delight.) So you're appreciating my true qualities—I *love* to be appre-ciated for *what I really am*.

The core "pathology"! "Don't be!" injunction versus a vital part of one's basic being which then turns against the self in *rage*.

Wants unconditional accept-ance of basic being.

V: Is something this hideous truly a part of me? Why me? Am I truly possessed? I'm just an ordinary good guy—I try to help people—how could something so hideous be a *part* of me?

D: You're all that great? You? You're a *nothing*. You're not worthy even to pick up the crumbs from under my table. Keep talking, whining, snivel-

"I'll be right there." Taken out of context, as it should be here, this is a positive statement. As the basic life force, a *hint* of the literal truth that, given permis-

ing—I'll be *right there* pushing you into the dirt!

V: How could I be singled out
for such a fate? What horrible thing have I done to deserve you?

sion to be, this will see the patient through thick and thin.

Patient (as victim) sees himself as
overly good (last statement) and
overly bad (here). Both have in
common *not real*. What *is* real
is disowned, and may reappear
as like a demon.

D: (Mocking.) You're just such
a pretentious little shit, but
you're really a nothing deep
down. You talk big, but you
have nothing to back it up.
I'm the one with all the
energy. All you're good for is
groveling at my feet.

V: What can I do to make you
go away?

D: Nothing, but I just love your
impotent struggling. (With
lip-smacking delight.)

(Break.)

V: Maybe I should integrate
with you. You may be evil,
but I'm going to *use* you for
my benefit. (Resolutely.)

D: *You're* going to use *me*??
(Sarcastic, sneering, condes-
cending.)

V: (Returning to frantic desperation.) What if I can't
stand it anymore and decide
to kill myself?

The big power play in the offing, the "victim" knows that at
least in this area, he has all the
cards.

D: What?? You?? You haven't
got the guts—anyway, your
lot in life is to grovel at my
feet, and I'm going to *keep*
you there! You *wouldn't dare*
try to get away from me—

A dangerous taunt. Some suicides may result from such an
intrapsychic transaction. *Thera-
apist should intervene directly*
here, if not sooner. He should
talk to the "demon" directly,

wherever you go, I'll hound
you forever!

validate the anger, and find out
how demon would have it if he
were to have everything his own
way. More often than not, the
requests are simple and of immense value to the overall Self.
Much of this bitter child–child
squabbling can be avoided by
the therapist, like a good parent,
talking to each part one-to-one,
after separating the combatants.

*V: You're the epitome of evil!
You have no right to exist!
Now that I know you're there,
I'm going to *destroy* you!!
You may think you're in con-
trol right now, but I'm going
to find some way to get rid
of you.

How would this feel to a small
child whose only sin is wanting
to live and who is too small to
express his needs in a more effective manner? Therapist can
make friends with Demon by
sharing this type of concern.

D: (Mocking, sneering.) Oh,
that's just music to my ears!
Keep talking—such *big* talk
from such a *little shit*.
(Laughs joyously, taking delight in his control.)

Used to lifelong abuse, will enjoy being alive "hell or high
water."

V: You Bastard!! Take that!!
(Kicks other chair forcefully
with his bare foot.)

D: (Taunting, mocking even
more.) How's the foot? Feel
real good?—Keep it up, old
boy—I'm right here, and I always will be.

Some of the worst intrapsychic
wars are *within* the Child ego
state.

(Break—Patient told that if he
simply continues the dialogue
change will happen by itself.

---

*A major shift: "Victim" is now expressing the destructiveness which was formerly
hidden behind the "helpless victim" position. Victim becomes a Persecutor. Neither
role is real living.

Returns to dialogue with more
confidence, but with bitter
vengefulness.)

V: I've told you once before and
I tell you again. I'm going to
use you for my benefit. (More
resolutely.)

D: You're going to use me?

V: If I kill myself, then I'll take   Literally true.
you with me.

D: I will have won then; you'll   A delusion shared by many
finally be out of your misery,   demons. Even in a non-multiple,
and I'll be free.   one ego state may perceive its
                                         existence as separate from an-
                                         other.

V: You'll be *free*? I will   The critical confrontation. This
have *destroyed* you,   is better done *by the therapist*,
totally—done—kaput! What   talking with the demon one-on-
kind of "freedom" is that for   one from a OK position. I have
someone who lives for the   yet to see a demon who will not
"sheer joy of living"? Maybe   cooperate. Not only does he
we should cut this bullshit   have his life at stake, but given
and start working together!   *permission to be,* he would like to
(Strong, confrontive parental   be a constructive part of a
manner.)   whole person.

D: (Thoughtfully, taking the   ". . . you've got a point there
matter into consideration.)   for a change." Demons accept
I've got to admit you've got a   this corrective feedback non-
point there, for a change.   defensively.
You seem to be getting some   "When you let your guard
strength, but don't worry—   down . . ." is, in itself, positive.
I'll be there waiting for you.   Let up on overcontrol and the
When you let your guard   life energy which is always there
down even just a little, even   is available to stand by and fuel
just a moment, I'll be there   the whole Self. "I'll be there."
ready to pounce upon you
and rub you back down into
the dirt.

V: Maybe—you're certainly evil

enough — but if I keep my
guard up, keep my strength
up, it's not going to be as
easy as before. Maybe you
had better play ball.

At this point, the demon may make his energy freely available to
the patient, who will then shift from being chronically depressed to
being quite energetic. The primary self, still somewhat split off from
— though not totally separated from — his demon, may still resist seeing the positive force in what had been disowned. At this point the
therapist may openly confront the negativity of the disowning in the
first place and establish increasing rapport with the demon. I believe
that this should usually come first — making an ally of what need not
have been a persecutor in the first place. I hope this becomes clearer
in the discussion which follows. While wars cannot always be avoided,
it is better to do so when possible — and it is possible far more often
than most of us realize.

REFLECTIONS ON GOOD AND EVIL

While we often colloquially refer to good and bad feelings, it is
more accurate to refer to these as pleasant or unpleasant. For no particular feeling, however disagreeable, is illegal, immoral or fatal. Nor
do I know of anyone who has been excommunicated from any church
because of his own private unpleasant feelings. I consider thoughts
subject to a negative value judgment only when they perpetuate undesirable outcomes that are not subject to voluntary control by the
central executive. To avoid the problems of a victim/demon split, we
need to be clear in our categories regarding where value judgments
are appropriate. They are appropriate without qualification only
toward outward behaviors.

Psychoanalysts like Kernberg (1975) and others describe one of the
defining characteristics of borderline patients as exaggerating within
themselves a split or dissociative barrier between what they perceive as
good and bad. In general, both poles of the good/bad split are so
overemphasized that they share one common feature — they are not
real. Whether good or bad at a given moment, the individual's sense
of real selfhood is distorted. Though what is perceived as good is often

in primary executive control most of the time, it may perceive itself as a victim of a demon, seen as a negative entity and hence suppressed. The demon then turns against the overall self sufficiently to validate the original derogatory value judgment, perpetuating a vicious circle.

At a social level, artificial separation of good and evil into separately existing spiritual forces or substances could be called moralistic dualism, a philosophical error possibly even more dangerous in social effect than the artificial separation of material and spiritual (ontological dualism) which I decried in *That Which Is* (1977a). If good and evil were truly separate and God only good, there would be no way out of the dilemma other than a bi-theism with a good god (God) and a bad god (Satan, the Devil). If this were an accurate perception, as still held by some religious believers, it would make sense to try to get rid of the evil, resulting in a crusader morality with the prime goal of fighting toward full extermination of evil so that a Utopian Good could triumph. The phenomenon of demonic possession at a psychological level can result from a personal belief in moralistic dualism.

If, instead, we assume that good and evil are not separate substances, but that both refer to inextricably interwoven aspects of existence, then the crusader morality takes on a less attractive color. If any entity or event has elements of both value poles, a conclusion I find hard to avoid, then abolishing the evil may also be destructive of vital aspects of existence and itself be evil. One cannot get rid of anything without destruction. If all that is is basically OK, a working principle, then the act of destruction is itself the evil. Within Christian theology, this position has been taken by Tillich (1951) and in psychoanalysis by Fromm (1973).

Underlying faith or the position of OKness of any person and all his parts is an understanding of polar opposites inherent in nearly every aspect of existence — All That Is as polarity. Any event can be seen in a good or bad light without violation of the data. A jar can be half full or half empty. By and large, the positive position feels better and works better. And it is far easier to achieve when value judgments are directed primarily to behavior as opposed to basic being.

The very act of trying to get rid of evil can, paradoxically, be what creates evil where it might not otherwise be. Hitler's Nazism and the Inquisition, among the most hideous of historical evil, are classic cases in point. The atrocities of the Inquisitors were reputedly carried out from a position of utmost religious righteousness with full intent to destroy evil, not recognizing the by-products as themselves evil. Nazism developed out of paranoid fear of Jewish and leftist elements which the Nazis then tried to exterminate, creating the worst holocaust in world history.

Mr. D in his victim polarity would be seen as resembling the inquisitor, wanting to destroy that part of himself that simply existed for the joy of existing. When the latter was seen as the positive entry it was, the problem progressed toward resolution.

An interesting twist in current theology is a tendency to look on such otherwise disagreeable concepts as "original sin" as a reflection of the good/bad split, with subsequent disowning of important parts of reality, therefore of God. Considered in this light, forgiveness is the process of letting go of that illusion and seeing what really is, not what we think it should be in terms of some limiting belief system. Its healing force is then a theological way of describing the acceptance of what was formerly considered demonic — forgiveness of the overall Self even more than the demon.

Within a given self the "demon" can be any drive which, instead of being accepted as a basic given of one's being, is defined as evil. In Freud's time, basic sexual drives were usually subject to this judgment, leading to the type of neurotic disorder described in much of his work. Today we are more likely to fear unduly aggressive drives. Looking objectively at both, it is not hard to see that behaviors arising from either of these two basic drive instincts can be good or bad at almost all levels, depending upon how they are expressed. The gratifying thing about making value judgments of behavior only is that it is precisely that area that can be changed in case of adverse judgment — changed, but not destroyed. Basic being is preserved, even enhanced. It can certainly work wonders to keep our categories clear.

Lowen (1967) succinctly summarizes the goal of therapy for the "possessed" patient as "Get in contact with the rejected body!" Humiston (1976) claims this is not enough, that it is necessary to experience *actually being* the demon as well, as Mr. D did so vividly in the encounter presented. Watkins (1978) formulates this as experiencing the demon as *subject* (me) instead of *object* (not-me). I believe that both processes must occur: 1) making friends of demons (as object), done both by the therapist and the patient's usual self, along with 2) re-owning the demon as subject.

While in the initial treatment of a severely dissociated individual the first process must usually precede the second, after this initial sequence both processes should repeat themselves so they can occur nearly simultaneously.

I suggest a fourfold maxim to summarize treatment of problems with demons:

1) Contact the demon (as object), validate its own needs and make an *ally* or friend of it.
2) Re-own that which had been dissociated away, and experience it as subject (me).
3) Accept, use and direct that energy of Self which had formerly been defined as evil.
4) Be in full control of this.

When this is accomplished, the patient is a whole person in the most positive sense. His full life energy is at his disposal and he is able to use it as he chooses.

CASE 2: PROTECTING THE TYRANT

A muscular young man, Mr. T, had carried a diagnosis of schizophrenia following a collapse of his real-life support system and subsequent suicide attempt, which led to hospitalization on a psychiatric unit. Not only did he manifest the psychomotor retardation of psychotic depression, behavior as if in slow motion, but he also reported hearing voices in his head running an almost continuous commentary on his worthlessness. "You're no good and would be better off dead — You can't succeed at anything, even suicide, but someday I'll manage to do it for you and put you out of your misery — Your feelings are stupid; you have no right to be angry when you're getting just what you asked for — You're simply no good, period. There's no value at all in even existing," etc., etc., etc. *ad nauseam*.

Mr. T appeared unreceptive to all manner of corrective feedback. He would at times make urgent demands on doctor and staff alike and blame them with hostile threats — not only when his demands were not met, but also when they were. At times he would be immobile, almost mute. At other times, he would become agitated and even threaten violence. At still other times, he would utter grisly comments on death, destruction, blood, and gore with a twinkle in his eyes that seemed not only incongruous but terrifying to many of his caretakers. His behavior seemed scrambled and apt to change for no apparent rhyme or reason.

Though not entirely unresponsive to antipsychotic medication, this man required massive doses of sedation when agitated. While experiencing, as a result of medication, some relief from his hallucinations, he was also extraordinarily sensitive to neurological side effects, giving his physician the sensation of walking a tightrope. At times he would appear sufficiently stabilized for release back into the community, although he soon decompensated again to the point of a return to the hospital, usually after a nearly lethal suicide attempt. He cooperated with treatment sometimes; at other times he would turn on the treating personnel for no apparent reason. At times he required involuntary commitment because he was a danger to himself.

When I first saw him, Mr. T presented his problem so clearly and lucidly that, following the same train of logic as with Mrs. R, I felt I would be well-advised to reconsider the diagnosis of schizophrenia. He manifested extreme incongruity in words and behavior with sudden switches in both and had nearly continuous auditory hallucinations of an extremely self-castigating nature. Yet, at no single moment was there any clear loosening of associations, the hallmark of schizophrenia. Although secondary symptoms were present in abundance, the primary 4 As of Bleuler (1911)—loosening of association, flattening of affect, autism, and social and emotional ambivalence were missing. Also, the hallucinations were *coherent* voices, themselves lacking any evidence of loose associations.

After a period of testing the growing therapeutic relationship, the patient was reluctantly willing to allow me to contact and talk with that part or aspect of himself that was finding expression through the voices, though he was far from convinced that this was not some malevolent external spiritual force similar to his father.

Identifying his usual self as T_1, I will refer to this other part as T_2. T_2 has actually given himself a different first name, without prompting or explanation. T_2 remained true to himself in telling me some of the negative things about T_1 that the latter had been hearing in his voices for nearly two horrible years. His name and personality were different, and the staff now recalled the patient's having occasionally called himself by a different name when in an apparently different state of mind. T_2 claimed to be entirely aware of all of T_1's behavior and experience, while T_1 was aware of T_2 only through hallucinations perceived and halfway conceived as external.

I made a tentative diagnosis of dual personality. This seemed to fit the data as well as schizophrenia—better actually, as neither part-self on its own showed classic thought disorder.

T_2, the one doing the talking in the hallucinations, was definitely a secondary personality—and a persecutor, as had been Mr. D's "demon" prior to therapeutic integration. But there was a difference. Most demons have been full of life energy in my experience, usually willing and able to become positive parts of a greater whole once their own existences were validated and their needs met. Not so with T_2. If anything, this part of the patient's psyche not only was both depress*ive* in fact and depress*ing* in effect, but also appeared even more depress*ed* than the primary T_1. When asked what would happen to himself (T_2) if T_1 were to succeed in killing himself and how he would feel about it, his replies were nearly opposite those of most demons.

First, there was not even an initial lack of awareness that if T_1 goes, T_2 goes with him. Second, he could not have cared less. "I'm not any good either. I try to keep him in line but it's impossible. He's no good, I'm no good, and I doubt that anybody or anything is all that great. I'd be just as happy as he to be out of my misery, and if I can help him or make him do it (suicide), I will do so any way I can." This was uttered in a flat, monotonous voice, with a rigid negative pseudo-parental content immovable to feedback.

Third, unlike most demons and other alter-personalities, T_2 was unconvinced about the desirability of seeing himself as a separate personality. Resistance to a diagnosis of dissociative disorder is common in a terrified primary, but rare with the secondary, who is usually all too eager for a chance to take over and come out. T_1 saw T_2 as a separate; T_2, while appearing immovable in his rigid negativity, evinced some of the usual psychiatric concerns about not wanting to do anything to worsen the split.

I thought to myself, none of this fits. Where's the life energy? It must be here somewhere or he would long since be dead. Are there more than two parts here? Is this a multiple, not simply a dual personality? How can I make contact with the life energy, wherever it is, that wants for himself not only life, but success in more than suicide? Or, as T_2 himself says, is there little point in doing anything? Is he simply a resistant psychotic depressive who probably will eventually suicide? Although he has made many nearly lethal attempts and certainly has the ability to succeed if that is his true intent, something always saves him.

What is that "something," I wondered, and how could I access it and make friends with it? Since this T_2 seems so negative, could I get rid of him? And should I do so, as Allison suggests? That trick smile Mr. T sometimes came up with when discussing something morbid looked like a child with something up his sleeve. Somewhat like a demon, it was in itself positive. Although he relaxed and mellowed briefly when I commented that the smile did not look all bad to me — about all the evidence I had of being seen and heard — no other demon would come out.

Whether or not such observations comprised the entire evidence, they were sufficient. I was being seen and heard by something like a scared child within the patient, even though virtually all communication with this part remained indirect until after the major therapeutic transactions. Further evidence, profound when viewed from a psychoanalytic perspective, was the forming of an intense, though quite unreal, type of emotional bond with and dependency upon myself. T's behavior increasingly manifested what Kohut (1971) termed narcissistic transference. While he idealized me, some part could always be accessed (sometimes T_2, other times not clear) that degraded me. At times he seemed to use me as a mirror of his perceptions and misperceptions of himself. When speaking of himself, he remained negative; when talking about me and certain therapeutic staff members, it was more often an unnaturally idealized positive. There was his positive part, or one of them, although it would show itself only when projected onto another person and seen as object.

The above was in some ways a "false positive," however — as unreal in its overidealizing as in its rigid self-degrading, though feeling better and accomplishing more when idealizing than when degrading. Bit by bit there evidenced an aspect of the patient more like an objective scientist or impartial observer. Despite the positive transference, whenever this newly accessed aspect could be contacted, descriptions of me were in such agreement with stark reality that neither I nor my colleagues could refute them. Even at the height of the narcissistic transference distortions, I was seen, in all my positives and negatives, as I actually am. For the most part, transference dominated the behavior of this man, who for a while would even decompensate and end up hospitalized whenever I was away on vacation or business, even though my style is to avoid such dependency whenever possible.

Mr. T gave himself increasing permission to use his intellectual curiosity to great effect in devouring any information relating to himself, as long as it was sufficiently neutral to be looked upon as objective, like a hobby, so to speak. I provided him with considerable informative material on dissociative disorder, which he critiqued at a very high level. While I object strenuously to Steiner's abuse of the term "pig" (1979), the patient saw in this concept a mirror of his own persecutory hallucinations — the still refractory T_2 who, despite considerable contact, remained as rigid and intractable as ever. When I shared my own concern over Allison's attempt to get rid of persecutors, the patient suggested on his own that to neutralize them would be equally effective without the implicit destructiveness that could itself become a problem.

T_1 found an ally in Steiner, and considerable symptomatic improvement occurred. I now had an interestingly dual professional relationship with the patient. At one level I was a psychoanalyst, with a patient in the throes of a dependent, narcissistic transference which was idealizing, subtly degrading and very much like a mirror of his self-misperception. At another level I was teacher and colleague, sharing objective information with him and subjecting it to mutual scrutiny in a much more symmetrical way. In this role he was able to take in the information that, not only with himself but also with external love objects, he simultaneously overidealized and degraded, both having a non-real quality in common. While we were talking superficially at a colleague-colleague level, several relaxed deep breaths indicated that he was taking this in at a very deep level and that it would have some impact, though what the impact would be was not yet certain.

Mr. T was again admitted to the hospital in crisis. While he had been episodically agitated throughout his disorder, this time was different. He was behaving like a cornered animal, fighting with every ounce of energy for pure survival. He was terrified and the thought content of his panic was overtly delusional. There was still no loosening of associations and his train of thought, though desperate and unrelated to current reality, was coherent. He was disoriented to time, consistently giving an exact date several years earlier, not long before his first suicide attempt and hospitalization. Was this a spontaneous hypnotic age regression, like that of Mrs. R, but to a time of perceived threat to life? At the time this question was not of relevance. This patient was desperate, threatening to do anything and beat down anyone in his way to escape his "persecutor." The only priority now was protection — forceful protection by whatever means necessary to ensure no harm to himself or others. Seclusion, massive sedation, restraints — all were used. There was no talk of the "I'm-only-trying-to-help-you" type, but simple firm repetitive assurance that he would be made safe, backed up by all the power at our disposal.

Here, undisguised at long last, was the part of Mr. T with all the life energy. Pure terrified child — terrified of total annihilation. It was not too difficult to see why the "healthy part" — which I assume was responsible for flashing the trick smiles — would never voluntarily come out. But here it was — out and desperate.

When the patient was quieter, but with no change in ego state, I asked him who he was; he replied with the name identified here as T_2. T_2 — the same part that had seemed like nothing but a depressed parent introject or "pig"? It seemed inconceivable that the part of this patient who had denied any value in life for himself or T_1 was now fighting for his life. So, is a depressed, primitive, and ineffectual parent figure identical in being to a terrified child? There are many theoretical issues and apparent contradictions here, which I will only begin to explore later.

Professional consultation was obtained from an expert in multiplicity. His diagnosis fit mine: definite multiple personality. In addition to providing forceful protection by any means, I was advised to assure the patient first of all that the creator is stronger than the createe, meaning that his persecutor, as a createe, could be conquered. The consultant further suggested that a latent ego state, if in danger, could be advised to rescue Mr. T by causing a hysterical immobilization. The patient accepted this with considerable relaxation.

This crisis appears to have been the decisive turning point, comparable to the initial 20 minutes with Mrs. R. It ended the psychotic episodes as well as massive dependency on medication, the hospital and me. As with Mrs. R, this was not "cure" in a characterological sense but simply approached cure at the more desperate psychotic and suicidal level. Mr. T was not entirely free of occasional splitting, even as manifested by episodic hallucinations, though these became far more benign and hardly an issue. Similarly, we were now seeing an immature personality in an adult body—as Mr. T himself readily acknowledged—exuberant and energetic, often nearly hypomanic. In this state he was like an integrated demon. There are other facets to his personality omitted here for the sake of simplicity.

What is striking is the continued emphasis that what was first a tyrant, behaving like a Steiner pig, was really the same as the desperate terrified child who finally had to be protected by whatever means. And this same child, when made safe, behaved like Mr. D's demon once the latter had been welcomed into the whole self.

Treatment was aimed not at getting rid of or even neutralizing the tyrant—but at making him feel safe.

The case of Mr. T, like many similar though less striking ones, raises many questions:

1) Is the tyrant, like many real-life tyrants, really a scared child underneath? If so, why does he not own up to it at the outset and seek protection?
2) Was there a further split within T_2, between the hypercritical tyrant and that which was being bullied—a dual personality within what already was only a part-self?
3) Did and do ego state boundaries shift, at the convenience of the moment?
4) Why did T_2, despite initial overall negativity, express realistic concern about exaggerating the already-existing split?
5) To what extent is a tyrant like T_2 an introject of a bad parent, and how much is it a reflection of the patient's own autonomous self?
6) Are Parent ego states separate entities introjected from perception of external parent figures and then personified, as implied by Berne's (1961) "exteropsyche," or are they aspects of the organism's own autonomous being?
7) Is a "narcissistic self-object" (seeing another person as a projection of a part of himself), as seen in Mr. T's transference and many dysfunctional love relationships, simply like an alter-personality projected into the perception of an external object?

8) Is working through a protracted transference neurosis a necessary and unavoidable part of treatment? If not, when can it be short-circuited and when not?
9) Is reparenting, to a degree present in all long-term therapy, necessary and desirable to make up for what a patient never had? Or can it lead to further undermining of the patient's autonomy, create further unnecessary dependency with its corollary risks, and even delay recovery and growth? Either and/or both? When?

I can touch here upon only those issues I see as global and encompassing a wide range of therapeutic dilemmas.

INTERNAL PARENTING AND TRANSFERENCE

To take charge of a symptom so that it becomes a skill was as much a treatment goal for Mr. T as it had been for Mrs. R, as described in Chapter 3. As with Mrs. R, this was but a prelude to a long process of maturation and growth beyond the scope of this inquiry. Even this initial phase, however, hardly required only 20 minutes. It lasted over a year and tested not only the patient's resources but my own and those of hospital staff and the patient's loved ones. This is more the rule than the exception in multiple personalities, even though the basic principle remains the same. It is easy to see why this is so from a close look at this particular case. The "symptom" referred to was not a simple process, as with Mrs. R, but was itself a complex of symptoms reflecting a disorder pervading his entire inner orchestra at many levels. The common denominator was a disorder in functions that we often call parental.

When one views an individual as a complex of many component parts, it is apparent that internal "parenting" is done by those ego states which serve both nourishing and limit-setting (regulatory) functions for other ego states and the overall self. This is the Parent of transactional analysis.

Most of the issues posed following the case presentation are far from resolved and are left open to stimulate further thinking. There are two, however, that merit further discussion in the context of this inquiry, those most relevant to what can make the therapeutic process more rapid, effective and safe: 1) When internal nourishing and limit-setting functions are disturbed — either inadequate or excessive and overly rigid—how can this imbalance be corrected optimally toward the goal of a spontaneous yet disciplined whole, where all parts find expression—without reparenting? 2) Are there any short-cuts to the prolonged working through of a transference that is still the cornerstone not only of psychoanalysis but of most long-term therapies?

I do not fully understand why some of my patients have developed intense narcissistic transference that required working through, and others not, however similar the nature and severity of their disorder; I suspect a skilled psychoanalyst might immediately observe certain psychodynamic differences. Subsequent developments in the case of Mr. T, where the transference was intense, difficult and fairly pro-longed, make it clear that the "healthy part" I had correctly assumed was there would not come out, despite encouragement by all means at my disposal, because it did not feel safe enough to do so overtly. It came out indirectly instead by way of the transference. When finally feeling safe, the patient could free himself sufficiently to move on with the business of life.

It follows that those cases in which transference was avoided, where difficult aspects could be dealt with more directly, were those whose part-selves felt secure enough to come out openly much earlier in therapy, instead of manifesting themselves only indirectly. While the dynamics of why this is so are not clear, it may have been in cases in which my own covert ego states were sufficiently resonant with those of the patient that therapeutic permission and protection were given and received beyond conscious effort or awareness of either party (Watkins, 1978).

Whether or not Mr. T's positive life energy part was so severely frightened that no manner of positive therapist behavior could have avoided the indirect route, by transference and its working through, is unclear. It is exactly here where I see the therapist's burden to be. His job is not to do for a patient what he alone can do for himself, but to resonate sufficiently with all the patient's aspects so that treatment can be a fully collaborative endeavor from the outset, obviating the need for either resistance or transference as understood by psycho-analysts.

This is a restatement of the first part of Erickson's maxims cited earlier. Instead of expecting the patient to speak the therapist's language, which most human beings would fight with all their might at some level, the therapist should speak the patient's language and join his system to gain rapport. To what extent this is possible I am not sure, recognizing that even if it is fully achieved, psychoanalysis would not become obsolete. It has been and remains one of the most potent research tools available for exploring the inner mind, though effective treatment can hopefully be accomplished more effectively by other means, as Freud himself hoped with equal sincerity.

Kohut (1971) and Kernberg (1975) have sparked new life into the psychoanalytic movement by discovering that, contrary to Freud's belief, narcissistic and borderline personalities are not necessarily unable to form a transference, therefore being unanalyzable. They do form intense transference relationships. Kohut terms these either "mirror," as a reflection of disowned aspects of primitive self-perception projected onto the analyst, or "idealizing," seeing the analyst as an idealized primitive parent. Both reflect aspects of the patient's self, as opposed to the neurotic transference described by Freud (1916), which referred more to early object relations. And both aspects of narcissistic transference are usually present and interwoven. As the patient overidealizes as well as degrades himself in a borderline good/bad split, one or more aspects of this unreal self-misperception will be projected onto his feelings toward and beliefs about his analyst. As with transference in general, this brings the problem into the here and now, where it can be worked through and resolved.

Following Kohut's lead, most psychiatrists now accept that narcissistic and borderline disorders are among the few remaining indications for formal psychoanalysis, the definitive treatment. Yet I doubt that Kohut himself would claim that it is the sole possible treatment, any more than Freud would have said hypnosis could never be of value. Kohut succinctly stated the goal of treatment as a change from pathological to healthy narcissism, with no attempt to get rid of it or to transform it to object relations.

This sounds to me like a different way of propounding my own dictum that our goal is to assist the patient in converting what was once a symptom into a skill. Since Kohut makes it clear that his own particular way of accomplishing his goal, though not necessarily the only way, is through psychoanalysis, his contribution stands out as a shining light, not only in that area but also in psychotherapy in its many forms. Information Kohut has supplied is not the exclusive property of psychoanalysts, but is in the public domain for therapists to use, add to and elaborate upon, each in his own unique creative way. Any one of the case histories presented here provides empirical data in support of the contention that formal psychoanalysis is not the only way a narcissistic patient can reclaim mental health.

One reason usually offered in support of psychoanalysis as the only definitive treatment is the assumption that the patient's ego structures or basic coping mechanisms are so defective that only repetitive contact over time can build what was missing. Although psychoanalysts respect their patients' integrity, knowing that only they can do their own changing and growing, that persistent negative implication of defect also underlies reparenting paradigms, in which values are imposed from without in order to provide what is assumed missing.

I take issue with that assumption. To begin with, an implicit as well as explicit insinuation that he is "defective" is so unpleasant to the patient that it may lead to seemingly insurmountable resistance. If an alternative viewpoint is justifiable, it may feel better and therefore work better. Enter the hidden observer as that alternative. That even the most disturbed of borderline cases may have intact hidden observers who can become internal self-helpers, as hinted in Hilgard's research, is a premise extended into the realm of dissociative disorder by Watkins and Allison, supported by Braun's work with super-multiples who are likely to be the same psychiatric entity as borderlines.

Taking this seriously, our job changes from needing to repair a so-called defect where none actually exists to finding the missing piece, accessing and empowering it, and helping the patient strengthen weak or frightened aspects for healthier living. If this can be done by the hypnotic equivalents I have been advocating, the psychoanalytic method is not necessarily so much wrong as inefficient. What might be wrongful, however, is discounting the patient's assets and the therapist's assumption of too much of the burden.

Hidden observers suggest an interesting twist on psychoanalysis and dissociation. Iatrogenically creating a multiple (here dual) personality may not be as much a risk of hypnotic therapy as it is an inevitable by-product of any treatment method where the incognito position of the therapist leads to displacement of the early life dilemmas onto what now is the transference. There are now literally two personalities. The primary self, in executive control and out for public view, is in the throes of a transference neurosis; behind a one-way amnesic barrier is the hidden observer.

Or was this transference/observer split present in some form even before treatment? If so, almost any neurotic problem coming to an analyst's attention could be considered dissociative disorder. I actually do believe this is the case in many senses. The hidden observer was then just as split off from power for action before as after development of the transference, and no modification of psychoanalytic theory would be needed — at the level of the executive ego state.

Here the psychodynamics of neurosis and transference would be little different from the way they are described by Freud and more recently modified by Kohut. What is new is simply the awareness of a hidden observer's presence. The present task is to empower it to take much of the therapeutic burden off the clinician, enhancing the patient's autonomy as well as facilitating therapeutic change.

In this light, another interesting twist is that failure to respect a patient's autonomy is the very criticism that long-term therapists of many persuasions have often leveled at hypnotists, along with a questionable assumption that change is not "real" change unless it takes lots of time and effort. Analysts often avoid giving therapeutic directives or using hypnotic techniques because they correctly want to avoid interfering with the patient's autonomy.

In my opinion this is the wrong decision but for the right reason — with reversal of categories. Only over a long period of time is there a danger that some of the values of any therapist will be introjected by a patient. Precisely because of the briefness of hypnotic and strategic interventions, their practitioners must respect the patient's integrity, for the only way to achieve results in a truly brief therapy context is when positive change grows out of the patient's intrinsic assets.

Hypnotists from Freud to the present know that pure direct suggestion rarely has more than a transient effect, except where the dynamics have been outgrown and the symptom persists as a habit only, which is not the case with multiple personalities. The challenge is to give a suggestion or directive that will not only access formerly hidden parts, but also prompt the patient to make changes which must still occur in his own way. Absolutely all the brief therapist can do is to change the frame of reference, usually by the "gentle art of reframing" (Watzlawick, Weakland and Fisch, 1974). This may accomplish as much as years of psychoanalysis. There is no way that change can be other than the patient's autonomous act.

CASE 3: A PARENT GROWS UP

Mrs. P sought treatment for chronic depression, difficulty with intimate relationships and episodic bouts of alcohol abuse. She was attractive, vivacious, quite receptive to insight and of fairly solid moral character. Rarely permitting herself to have fun, she would episodically cut loose during a drinking episode. It was clear that she victimized herself with a rigid, punitive tyrant, not unlike that of Mr. T. Though this was at the ego state level, as opposed to an alter-personality, she suffered under its tyrannical regime.

But Mrs. P was perplexed. "How," she wondered, "could this be when I had no such critical parent in real life? With absolutely no limits or control placed upon me, I could do virtually what I wanted as far back as I could remember." When I asked how it would feel to a tiny child not to have any limits placed upon her behavior, she responded tearfully, "Not very safe — really scary, in fact." Was it possible that she had created that tyrant herself as a primitive internal parent to provide the missing control and safety? That supposition was met with an affirmative response of tearful relief.

Since a small child is intellectually incapable of distinguishing between the categories of basic being and behavior, it may be unnecessary to go further in uncovering the origin of error in making judgments against one's basic being, instead of one's behavior. People with this disorder, almost uniformly exhibiting some degree of narcissism, have developed their internal parenting difficulties at so early an age that complete avoidance of that critical philosophical error would have been virtually impossible.

After simple discussion of this perspective at an informational level, Mrs. P was able to assess her own needs as an adult woman and update her internal parenting to suit her current needs. The first step was to give herself permission to have fun without getting intoxicated, which she was able to do remarkably easily, to her own amazement. Her depression gradually lifted and she was able to enter and eagerly pursue an educational program, doing well at my last contact with her.

This and similar cases suggest that the parents within are not always simply introjects of original parent figures. That different siblings may have entirely different internal parenting in spite of sharing real parents also suggests more creativity on the part of the individual child than pure passive incorporation. Yet creativity does not arise out of a vacuum, of course, and a creative child, like any artist, must use whatever material or information is at his disposal. Since that for developing parental functions is mainly input from parents, it is not difficult to see why most internal parent ego states resemble the actual parents upon whom they were modeled.

Even with perceptions known not to be passive incorporations but creative actions, the concept of "introject" can have only relative philosophical validity — basically, in the realm where it proves useful. Not only did Mrs. P transgress beyond those limits of relevance, but so too do all imaginary playmates who serve self-nurturing functions without significantly resembling actual parent figures. That we can easily create them without extended reparenting is a datum I cannot emphasize too strongly.

The human organism has a remarkable capacity for creating that derives from one's life energy aspects. Powerful parent-like entities can be created by a simple act of imagination. In treatment this can be assisted by hypnotic imagery. It is little different from the process of a child's creating an imaginary playmate, as so lucidly described by Pines (1978). If this new part of him serves a parenting function that both feels and works better, it may become cathected with sufficient psychic energy to become a major ego state in its own right, just as an imaginary playmate can sometimes become an alter-personality. Such internal parents may bear little resemblance to either the patient's actual parent figures or to his therapist, having been tailored to fit that individual's unique needs. And who can know these needs better than the patient himself? Especially vital is his all-knowing unconscious — a force I suspect is behind creative hypnotic imagery, as well as dreams.

Mrs. P illustrates how this ability has been used creatively to provide protection for herself as a child, in the only way a small child knows when external parental controls are inadequate. As an adult, it became maladaptive — a symptom. Using the same ability by which she had originally developed her tyrant, she was able just as easily to update her internal parenting to serve the needs of an adult woman better. It was now a skill of the highest order.

Even a seemingly rigid and limited ego state can reveal within itself the paradoxical elements and polar opposites we know we must look for in whole organisms. While we do not understand ego state reversals, their occurrence is nothing new to experienced hypnotists or hypnotic subjects who utilize this phenomenon frequently in their work. Just as a real-life bully is often a scared child in need of protection, who will stop persecutory behavior once he feels safe, this is true of bully-like tyrant ego states as well. Just as healthy children, so much in need of nourishment, are often the best at giving it when their own needs are met, a free child ego state, given permission to exist, can often serve as a self-nurturing parent far more effectively than any introject.

Certain polarities seem to go hand in hand. I hope I have illustrated some of the most important and commonly occurring paradoxes in the three cases presented. What seemed demonic proved to be pure life energy, appearing persecutory only when persecuted. When given permission to be, it was not only a free child in need of being cuddled, but also best able to do the cuddling. When excessively critical behavior is seen, it often works better not to take arms against the persecutor but to call forth his softer side, comfort the scared child beneath the critical behavior and provide protection. When self-nurturing behavior seems absent, we can often find the potential for creating it within the very part that seems to need it most.

All can be reduced to a common denominator, the Big P — Permission to Be. Freeing the potential inherent in basic being usually involves changing one's frame of reference. This — more than getting rid of what somebody cannot rid himself of or trying to add what nobody but a given individual can create for himself — is ultimately what most often proves therapeutic.

The structural issues raised by ego state reversals can only be posed for further study. Do they reveal further splits within an ego state or are they aspects of just one? Do ego state boundaries shift to suit the needs of the moment? Can old ego states grow up or are they replaced by new ones? I suspect the answers can be either/and. While the theoretical questions are intriguing, what matters most to the clinician is how to utilize what we observe to our best advantage without having to understand what we may never fully understand. It is this propensity with which hypnotherapists have become most comfortable as well as skilled, working as they do with a phenomenon they understand no more than does anyone else. Awareness of the polar elements in any entity or event is what underlies the power of positive reframing, so that a simple shift in our frame of reference may nullify old rigidities, allowing life to move ahead.

8

Disorders of Extension and Expansive States

At the other end of the unity and multiplicity spectrum from dissociation, upon which attention has been focused so far, is what I refer to as extension or expansion. By this I mean the process in which an individual's sense of selfhood extends beyond his physical boundaries so that he experiences as self what is actually beyond.

Like dissociation, extension occurs at all levels along a continuum. At the simplest level are empathy and identification, both well defined in psychiatry as providing a link between self and others. Certain religious or spiritual states of mind, experienced as a oneness with nature or with God, occur at levels from the simplest to the most sublime. That one can take normally unconscionable risks to self and loved ones in time of war testifies to an extension of selfhood to society, at least at some level.

At the extreme end of the extension continuum is what I refer to as a *symbiotic psychosis*, where a patient's sense of boundary between himself and non-self is so blurred that reality-testing becomes impossible. Like major dissociation, even this degree of extension may at times have a healthful context, occurring in love, hypnosis and the religious experience (Beahrs, 1977a). And again, effective treatment

166

philosophy should be discovering how to remove the phenomenon from the realm of psychopathology and use it adaptively.

Any definition of disorders of extension is necessarily less precise than is the case with dissociation and its vicissitudes, for language, both written and spoken, is by nature dissociative in its tendency to compartmentalize and label entities and combine them into patterns. It is therefore less suited to discussing an expansive process whereby things become less compartmentalized and boundaries blurred.

Another effect of this limitation of language in connection with disorders of extension is that patients whose problem is at this level are even more likely than multiple personalities not only to be perceived as, but actually to be, psychotic in not being able to share the agreed-upon realities upon which most people base their lives.

Like the hypnotized subjects I consider their healthy equivalents, individuals with problems in their sense of unity and multiplicity both dissociate and extend simultaneously. A simple case example from the arts will illustrate what is happening and lead to a more formal discussion of disorders of extension.

THE NARCISSISTIC SELF-OBJECT AS A PROJECTED ALTER-PERSONALITY

In the case history of Mr. T, it will be recalled that a most significant part or aspect of the patient first "came out" not overtly, but in disguised form in what is generally called a narcissistic transference. Through it he perceived me, his therapist, not as he customarily would but as a projection of parts of himself he refused to own up to as his own. This phenomenon is well-known to any modern psychoanalyst. I am mentioning it again not only for the theoretical interest of taking a new twist on a familiar phenomenon, but also because the misery to all concerned arising from dysfunctional love relationships so fits the paradigm. How much of this suffering can be avoided by preventive psychiatry and how much is part of the basic human condition I still wonder. The human condition is sometimes defined as the struggle to find "meaning in life," which seems also to be a part of the narcissistic dilemma.

That the librettists of Grand Opera felt narcissistic disorder and the human condition were one and the same is clear to anyone familiar with a sufficient number of opera scripts. In my estimation, well over 80 percent could be a verbatim case history from the investigations of Heinz Kohut! Nowhere is this life tragedy exemplified more explicitly and movingly in its full horror than in the libretto of the opera *Carmen*. The protagonist is not Carmen herself, who appears incapable of any kind of meaningful love. It is Don Jose, an intense, passionate and dutiful young soldier who cannot let go—first of his mother, then of his duty and finally of Carmen.

We might ask what it was at a deeper level that he could not let go of. The psychoanalytic answer might well be an idealized mother-image not sufficiently separated from his perception of himself. What Don Jose would not let go of, then, was something inextricably associated with himself and preserved with the full force of the survival instinct, leading to his slaying Carmen out of desperation over her having rejected a love never there from the start. The context of Carmen and Jose's union is clear enough to overrule any possibility of real love on the part of either. It is even questionable whether there had been sexual consummation. Carmen was simply there at the right time to serve as a projection screen for a vital aspect of Jose's basic being—probably the feminine anima part he could not confess to with his hyper-masculine exterior, though it was what he most needed.

As a paradigm of narcissistic personality disorders, Don Jose illustrates another facet of unity and multiplicity as we see it in psychopathology. He both dissociates and extends, in a way in which the two are inseparably interwoven and a manifestation of the same process—and in this particular case most dysfunctional. His sense of cohesive self is not sufficiently stable, his ego boundaries unclear and his perception of Carmen not that of a separate person but an extension of himself. He is "extended" in the sense of his selfhood's going beyond his body to what was actually a Jose-Carmen symbiosis—most likely a reenactment of what Don Jose never resolved between himself and his mother. His self went beyond, then, though hardly in a functional way.

But as a projection of a disavowed part of Don Jose representing the ideal feminine, Carmen represents a vital though disowned aspect of his existence, which might have appeared as a demon in a case like Mr. D's. Carmen did behave demonically and she paid the price.

When she betrayed Don Jose, it was as if the most vital part of himself was gone. Yet all he killed, psychologically, was a projection.

That Carmen is among the most popular of all operas testifies to how much most people can relate to this anguish, an understanding of which can reveal a vital lesson of life and love.

EXPANSIVE PERSONALITIES

Mrs. E, a rather pathetic-appearing middle-aged woman, was well-known not only to me but to à large number of mental health personnel from past contacts. Frail and sickly, she was chronically and often psychotically depressed; her expressions of either anger or pleasure were no more convincing to herself than to others. She came across as both *sick* — medically and psychiatrically — and *empty* — a shell of a person. Her sole gratification was complaining about her misery, including numerous hypochondriacal symptoms and multiple ideas of persecution by those who had cared for her in the past.

Although I often became impatient with the persistence with which this woman refused to let go of the victim role at its worst extreme and often told her so without hiding my frustration, I could not help being moved by a certain aura of pathetic desperation and persistence. Mrs. E had this effect on several other therapists as well. Several of them gave unsparingly of their time to listen to what seemed to be an endless broken record. Something within Mrs. E was reaching out to and resonating with at least some therapeutic selves, though what that something might be did not become clear to me until later, following what was one of the most moving experiences in my psychiatric career.

Mrs. E, angry at the circumstances, was referred to me again for a routine examination. In some ineffable way she seemed stronger. "I've been talking to God the past few weeks," she explained. "He uses such big words that I have to look them up in the dictionary. Doesn't that sound crazy? But when I look them up, it always makes sense."

Here, talking with God — auditory hallucinations in a patient with a long history of schizophrenia, along with about every other category invented by modern psychiatry. Yet Mrs. E looked and acted less crazy than I had ever seen her. As I interviewed her now, she reported the commentary "God" was giving her, the vocabulary at a college-plus level. Even before she asked for definitions of relevant words, I recognized the content of her voice as exactly on target to an uncanny degree — not frightening in the least but strangely stirring, even comforting. The patient would comment upon the voice's assessment of what I, as therapist, was probably thinking and feeling at the time with such correspondence to my actual inner subjective state that it literally resembled pure mind-reading. When I occasionally had to check on a challenging word myself, the content remained precise.

By conversing with this God of Mrs. E's indirectly through her, I obtained a clear and coherent past history that had formerly eluded me, learning how after bitter life tragedy she had abdicated virtually her entire life force, leaving what indeed was just a shell of a personality. My reaction was a simple, heartfelt "Welcome back!" to which she responded appropriately. With careful history-taking, it became clear that in this patient's childhood she had done sufficiently wide reading that it was not necessary to speculate on supernatural intervention to explain her new large vocabulary and comforting affect.

The apparently near-perfect reading of my mind, not yet at all threatening, can be seen as RESONANCE in capital letters, for Mrs. E had certainly known me long enough to have learned my quirks and to be able to read and interpret my nonverbal communication. But with such pinpoint accuracy? And in a way containing not the slightest sense of threat? While she had been just like a shell for decades, the level of evolution this "expansive part," for want of a better term, had reached without ever being "out" was far beyond her premorbid personality. I am unwilling to speculate on all this except that what finally appeared, first as the "voice of God" and then as an extension of Mrs. E's sense of selfhood, pushed the limits of human capability as far as I can imagine their being pushed — not necessarily beyond, but certainly as far.

Helen Watkins (1980) cites the case of a rather negative "Woman in Black" who, when her needs were validated and negaive behaviors confronted by the rest of the patient's self, simply seemed to evaporate. In her place appeared a positive, nurturing, ideal mother-type "Lady in White." Asked where she came from she replied, "Beyond. . . ." My first assumption, in accord with accompanying discussion concerning this case, would be that the Lady in White was like a new nurturing ego state created by the overall self as an imaginary playmate, an approach I am suggesting become routine strategy in treatment. "Beyond" would then refer simply to having been created on the spot, not already there. *Or??* I do not know and prefer to keep an open mind.

In writing on dreams and the occult, Freud (1933) found that analysis of many ordinary dreams revealed latent content inexplicable short of telepathic thought transference. Especially interesting in his observation was the lack of any hint of such telepathy until the dream had been analyzed! What Freud could explain by no traditional scientific means was sufficiently modified by the patient's dream work so that it did not appear in the manifest content. The issue would never have been raised without analysis of the dreams—a reversal of the usual situation where extrasensory phenomena will not withstand analytical scrutiny.

No scientist or psychiatrist should ignore the work of Jane Roberts, a well-known "psychic" who writes books not only in her usual personality state, but even more frequently from an expansive one called Seth. In the latter case, books are verbally dictated by her as by Seth with booming voice and blazing eyes totally different from her still energetic usual self. Seth carries a slight to definite aura of the demonic. Roberts frankly admits in her writing to having had considerable emotional deprivation as a child, like Mrs. E, and the content of Seth is not unlike that of Mrs. E's God, only far more expansive. I find the Seth books, written in a Biblical style somewhat like "That is what is, and this what you need to do," remarkably nonthreatening in spite of my customary rebellious response to parental preaching.

Psychiatrically, the Seth phenomenon poses issues similar to those facing Mrs. E. After dictating as Seth, Roberts has partial to total amnesia for the content of the Seth sessions, although she can often partially recall the autohypnosis. Is she then a multiple personality, in whom the splitting enhances health instead of impairing it? Or is she truly a spokeswoman for a Spirit-guide extending beyond her body in both space and time? She herself is not fully satisfied with either point of view.

At another level is the content of the Seth books. In *The Nature of Personal Reality* (1974), Seth presents a systematic exploration of the effect of one's beliefs on creating one's own personal reality, and how to manipulate these to enhance one's healthful potential. While con-

taining some material that jars those of scientific persuasion, myself
included, this book nonetheless seems to me as to many others to surpass in quality anything extant in the current mental health literature!
Not only is the altered state of consciousness when Roberts becomes
Seth of interest to the psychiatrist, but the content of his productions
is equally absorbing. Further, speculations on the nature of physical
reality, with ideas on space and time wild and imaginative and far
beyond scientific testing, are exciting and stimulating to the creative
thinking of most readers.

I have recently taken several steps back from initial skepticism since
reading the work of David Bohm (1971), once a youthful colleague of
Einstein, who has published controversial views on the nature of reality designed to make sense of inherent contradictions between quantum and relativistic physics. His interpretations point in exactly the
same direction as those of Seth, who seemed to appear from out of the
blue—or beyond. Clearly something inexplicable yet important is going on.

Roberts' Seth books are all readily available for anyone to study and
attempt to explain and the Seth phenomenon and its content are in
the domain of world experience—but far beyond explanation. I am
inclined to take a cautious position in approaching expansive
phenomena of this type, merely wanting to emphasize that we can
and should no longer wish them away. As with psychiatric systems,
any world view may have its own limits of relevance. Ours are now being challenged.

HYSTERICAL PSYCHOSES

The topic of expansive personalities hits at the other end of the
unity-multiplicity continuum. While previous discussion has emphasized the dissociative aspect—when it is useful and when not to see
ourselves as composed of many part-selves like a multiple personality—
it is no longer possible to avoid an extensive aspect as well, concerning when it is useful and when not to perceive ourselves as parts of
greater whole. Neither Mrs. E's God nor Jane Roberts' Seth are simply
part-selves; they are far too expansive, more like entities extended
beyond the individual's usual bounds. With Mrs. E, those bounds had
become so constricted that she was simply re-owning her actual self,

first perceiving it as hallucination, albeit an expansive one. As indicated earlier, this pushes but does not transgress the limits of that interpretation.

In the case of Roberts, however, the expansiveness of her usual self seems to belie such a reading. And that Seth has expounded content attracting the serious attention of even some physicists is hardly to be discounted.

Mrs. H, a bright young lady with an inquiring mind and problems with relationships, came into my office in crisis. She had been experiencing bizarre changes in her body image and telepathic and clairvoyant thought content that she believed frequently checked out. She was terrified that she was or might be considered "crazy." Her thoughts at many levels did sound mad, though the experiences were very real and suggestive of spontaneous hypnotic behavior if considered apart from content. Mrs. H did not appear deranged, however; her usual state was already a somewhat expansive personality. I merely emphasized to her the distinction in categories between her experience, which in itself could be neither sane nor insane, and her thought content, which clearly could be psychotic if grossly contradictory to reality-testing as generally defined. In this particular case, my advice to take note of her experience with extreme caution against over-explaining it was sufficient to provide relief. To my knowledge, Mrs. H has had no psychotic breakdowns and has made considerable personal growth.

I have dealt with several patients of both sexes who have experienced similar phenomena but whose beliefs were far over the red line, their behavior sufficiently disturbed and disturbing to warrant psychiatric hospitalization. When seen by other psychiatrists, they have generally been diagnosed as schizophrenic. Although schizophrenia was indeed the closest approximation possible to a descriptive diagnosis using the old diagnostic manual (DSM-II), many psychiatrists, including myself, prefer a separate label, *hysterical psychosis*.

Described in some depth by Martin (1971) and others, it is usually an acute decompensation with loosening and dissolution of ego boundaries (pathological extension) and delusions that are wide and expansive with considerable emotional impact, though simply not standing the test of secondary-process logic. That this is a valid criterion for psychosis follows from the fact that past this point behavior usually becomes grossly maladaptive and inappropriate — not just because beliefs are out of line with sociocultural standards.

At times it is extremely difficult to exclude true schizophrenia, for the dissolving of ego boundaries can mimic the pathognomonic loose association of the schizophrenic. There are, however, several features distinguishing the hysterical or symbiotic psychosis from schizophrenia: 1) Verbal productions are expansive instead of limiting and not infrequently the patient will emerge from the psychosis at a healthier level than before. This fits the paradigm of spontaneous hypnotic trance behavior perceived by Frankel (1976) as a "coping mechanism." 2) Rarely is there a family history of schizophrenia, even though its familial and biochemical aspects are rapidly becoming better known. 3) Attempts at treatment with antipsychotic medication are often bitterly resisted and bizarre neurological side effects are more the rule than the exception. The psychotic episode usually follows a severe bind or life crisis and generally resolves on its own. The new manual, DSM-III, has at long last included hysterical psychoses, labeled "Brief Reactive Psychosis." Unfortunately, the manual does not distinguish these from schizophreniform psychosis or schizophrenia on the basis of the clinical features, but only on the duration of illness. In the same way that the diagnostic manual encourages overdiagnosis of schizophrenia at the expense of dissociative disorder, I believe it creates problems by failing to distinguish between the different types of psychosis on the basis of clinical features more refined than temporal duration of the episode.

Just as there is a continuum of dissociation from normal mood swings all the way to multiple personality, I would suggest there is a comparable continuum of extension starting with empathy and identification, then ranging from simple expansive spiritual-like states of consciousness to either a full-flown hysterical psychosis or a Seth-like phenomenon. They can be most dysfunctional or most valuable.

I would like to offer a comparable treatment paradigm. Instead of arbitrarily dubbing the psychosis "pathological," define it as a skill not currently being used to the patient's advantage. When the individual is psychotic, regressed primary process logic prevails at the expense of secondary process reality logic. Since the content of regressive thinking can be rich and symbolic, it is worth paying attention to. The goal then is not to be "cured" of a type of thinking that may be of great value, but to place it under secondary process scrutiny. We then have what Arieti (1976) calls tertiary process, the essence of creativity.

Dealing with severe recurrent hysterical psychosis can be as trying to the most skilled of psychotherapists as dealing with a multiple personality. This is not surprising since they are of the same nature of disorder, simply at different ends of a dissociation-extension continuum. Perhaps the biggest challenge for the therapist is speaking the patient's language, often a prerequisite for any type of rapport. This language is that of the dream world, or the unconscious, which all therapists share. The trick is for the therapist to slip into this level while retaining his own grasp of secondary process reality. In other words, he must become increasingly skilled at tertiary process in order to accomplish this safely.

I believe that autohypnotic experience, all of it tertiary process if under reality control, is invaluable for this purpose. The therapist first communicates at a primary-to-primary level that to an onlooker appears bizarre. As rapport is established, he may reply to a patient's symbolic communication with a symbolic one of his own. A relaxed smile by the patient indicates that he knows what is going on and is ready. When the patient discusses his experience with the therapist at a reality level, he is usually ready to leave the hospital.

In my opinion, a doctor should always take a desperate plea for no medication seriously, even more so when there is a report of side effects. Contrary to indicating that the patient "wants to stay sick," it is more apt to mean that medication is not indicated and may be a diagnostic clue to dealing, not with schizophrenia, but with a disorder of extension. In addition, it is important to pay close attention to symbolic and nonverbal communication. Ordinarily, when the symbols can be translated, as from dreams and mythology, as suggested by Jung (1964), the entire problem will be right on the table, so to speak. There are generally recurrent stresses. Identifying these and encouraging alternative coping methods may forestall future episodes.

It is also well to bear in mind that the "psychosis" may not be across-the-board. At times, the patient will be in an expansive mystic-like state with enhanced awareness and functioning, not unlike what occurs in mystics and those experienced with autohypnosis and varieties of meditation. He may be psychotic in only one or a few areas of life. If so, those particular ones are most likely the stress points or areas of vulnerability that mark the focal point of ongoing treatment. Clarification and simple feedback are often best here.

THE MYSTIC STATE

Expansive states of consciousness are prized and often sought by many individuals, especially within certain sociocultural frameworks. At times such a state can simply be respite from the demands of daily living. At others — in such extreme mystical states or religious experience as described by James (1902) — it can be a turning point in a person's life. As indicated above, consideration of these phenomena is more difficult than in the case of dissociation, because of the very nature of language.

Extending, a loosening rather than defining of boundaries among subject, object and different entities, is more capable of being felt or sensed than described linguistically. It may actually involve a shift to intuitive or primary process. Since this is far more flexible than secondary process, though less tangible, such a shift may explain the sense of expansiveness, as well as its experiential similarity to pure hypnosis or even hysterical psychoses. In fact, I can hardly find a definition of hysterical psychosis that goes beyond a positive expansive state of consciousness, except for delusional beliefs that contradict the evidence and get the patient into trouble.

Most prized worldwide of all normal expansive or extensive phenomena is the state of being in love. I have touched upon this earlier (1977a) and will elaborate further below. In likening love to hypnosis, Freud (1920) saw in both instances a merging of one's sense of self to include that of the love object. Sullivan defined love as that state in which the needs and welfare of the object are as important as one's own — perhaps even inseparable from them.

Freud astutely observed that love involves both a loosening and a strengthening of the sense of self. For there is a feeling of losing oneself in a greater self in the love union — an extension — while also gaining a stronger sense of personal potency as part of that union.

James describes the mystical experience in its most extreme form as having four qualities: 1) ineffability (beyond words — expansive, not dissociative); 2) a noetic quality, carrying a sense of intuitive knowledge so authoritarian as to feel like a divine command — a sense of authority that can make itself felt long after the state itself has passed; 3) transiency—of short duration, the mystic state itself rarely lasting more than a half-hour of clock time; and 4) passsivity—selflessness, as if the mind itself were held in abeyance by a greater power.

These qualities, shared to a degree by hysterical psychotics, people "delirious with love," and those who cultivate expansive states of consciousness, are not unfamiliar to hypnotists. In defining hypnosis as similar to love, Freud was referring to a letting go of one's usual self and expanding the ego so as to encompass both the hypnotic situation and the hypnotist.

A hypnotic suggestion can carry the same noetic quality described by James and also felt by one in love. Yet we have been working within a view of hypnosis defined more by Hilgard as comparable to dissociation. Are hypnosis and the gamut of healthy and less healthy mental phenomena likened to it dissociative as well as expansive? Is the hidden observer an extensive as well as dissociative phenomenon? This would fit the experience of expansive spiritual guide-type personalities like Seth and Mrs. E, as well as fitting Allison's distinctions between ISHs and pathological alter-personalities.

Further questions arise in this connection. Does useful extending enhance ability to dissociate creatively, thereby increasing power for action? And does useful dissociation comparably enhance one's ability to experience such expansive phenomena as love and the divine? Does hypnosis cover the gamut and are dissociation and extension perhaps in some way even one and the same, considered at a higher level?

I suspect the answers are all yes. But because of the ineffability of extension carried by the structure of thought and language itself, I do not feel able to describe or analyze the extensive pole with anything approximating the attention I have given the dissociative. I can only sense and intuit an area which, true to description by others, is both healthy and sometimes awesome or even painful. It feels more like a matter of faith than belief. For I have long believed there is more to life than what we can dissect and analyze and psychiatrize.

I hope this may allow the entire discussion to lead to a degree of closure emphasizing the need for some grounding in one's basic integrity. That this is ultimately far beyond any particular psychiatric, religious or philosophical belief system brings us back to the very root of healthful living itself—faith and commitment.

Epilogue:

Beyond Psychiatry

A comprehensive approach to mental health based on lack of formal theory and the security it provides presents the practitioner with a unique difficulty. Where do we take root? Upon what do we define basic values and structure so that what we do is not only flexible but also both competent and ethical? A theory without a theory, in essence what I am proposing, might be seized upon by advocates of the "flow with it" type of pop psychology in apparent justification of lack of structure, with results far from satisfactory to society at large. This is the last thing I would want to see happen.

While Erickson's (1976) familiar remark that there is "no place for theology in mental health" is not actually a misquote, it seems to me to run a critical risk of misplaced emphasis. The many in-depth discussions I was fortunate enough to have with Erickson revealed the vital point of this dictum—a context that can be ignored only at peril. We must reconsider distinctions between faith and belief, and between first-order Reality (All That Is) and the infinite number of finite second-order realities that portray but one aspect of this greater Reality. Any belief system or theory (the "theology" of Erickson, I feel sure) must have its limits of relevance. With the infinite complexity of dimensions in human life, the likelihood is minimal that any system (and I do not except my own) can adequately meet the needs of all patients.

To impose one particular system or "theology" is then truly inappropriate in mental health. It violates respect for the integrity of each unique human being. Yet it is only that respect — along with a therapist's willingness to adapt his own views to any particular situation — that can provide the awesome flexibility and therapeutic potency so characteristic of Erickson. He himself assiduously avoided forming a theory or system of his own as too limiting. Though far from discouraging many of his followers from thus conceptualizing his work, he usually emphasized that in so doing they were describing but one aspect of his work. The implication is that, like any theory, an "aspect" is limited and limiting, even if derived from an expansive body of work.

Reflecting upon Erickson's personal life, I find there a pervasive solidarity and integrity and a code of values respectful of that of every patient, whether or not this was apparent to them. Even when dealing with a multiple personality, he emphasized that each part must be treated with respect and dignity. His faith in all that is included all human individuals and all their parts as basically alright; his particular expertise lay in an ability to seek, find, and utilize this OKness wherever it seemed most missing. At this level is where "theology" is not only relevant but essential to mental health — what *Unity and Multiplicity* is all about.

From faith and an endorsement of all that exists, plus a humble awareness of the limitations of any of our beliefs, come both the roots of integrity, which give us an all-pervading feeling of strength and stability, and the flexibility of beliefs and their resulting methods that enhances our power for action. The one is extension at its best; the other, optimal dissociation. One depends on the other. Within the continuum of all that is, seen as polarity, each polar opposite needs the other, is attracted to it and is in some sense inseparable from it. This affinity between apparent opposites is another way of looking at the concept of love. Within the constraints of language, this is perhaps the closest we can come to describing the organizing principle of existence.

Expansive new works suggesting broad new vistas within physics, psychotherapy, and spirituality are not the only definitive statements on the limitation of our current fund of world knowledge, especially in psychiatry. Even the Golden Rule — "Do unto others as you would have them do unto you" — points beyond the limitations of current psychiatry, which so emphasizes working through one's own problems and meeting one's own needs. A commitment to something beyond oneself may not only be morally right, whatever that means, but may feel better and work better even for the self. As Freud said of love, an individual may lose himself, yet find himself again at a higher level. We need to transcend the pop psychotherapy "theology of self" as urgently for the sake of self as for others.

Now we can take delight in expanding our beliefs and extending our power for action, continually bearing in mind the necessity of our limitations — not as a threat but as reassuring. This in itself is much of the joy of life!

Appendix I:

Co-consciousness and

Psychic Uncertainty

I include this more detailed exposition as an appendix for those who would like an opportunity to study and critique the underlying logic of this work in more depth. Especially important is the A/ Not-A Absurdity, discussed in Chapter 2 of the text. Likened to a *Psychic Uncertainty Principle*, it is critical to an in-depth understanding of my theoretical position, which includes my rationale for avoiding overly precise theory. By discussing its ramifications in depth, I hope not only to win more serious consideration for the basic issues of *Unity and Multiplicity*, but also to offer psychic uncertainty itself as a principle having profound implications for theory far beyond the scope of this book. This discussion has been omitted from the text proper in the hope that what is already present is sufficient grounding in theory for the practicing clinician.

I will first attempt to define some basic terms used throughout the book and to show at the outset the difficulty in avoiding ambiguity, suggesting that "fuzzy" thinking may be unavoidable for the issues at hand — even in principle. This will include a statement of the underlying logic of my basic position, of co-consciousness, in its bare essentials. Then I will present an outline of the basic reasoning behind psychic uncertainty, whose relevance to the position of co-conscious-ness will already have been seen. Last but by no mean least are several examples from the medical and psychiatric profession illustrating how uncertainty and imprecision not only are unavoidable, but at some level may actually enhance our understanding and power for action.

DEFINITIONS

Co-consciousness

I define this term as "the existence within a single human organism of more than one consciously experiencing psychological entity, each with some sense of its own identity or selfhood relatively separate and discrete from other similar entities, and with separate conscious experiences occurring simultaneously with one another within this human organism."

So defined, co-consciousness denotes what is actually the thesis of the entire book. We are not just a cohesive self, but also a composite of many aspects, facets, or parts which have their own personalities and ongoing experience simultaneous with one another and with the overall self. Likening the whole mind to a group of individual people, each part has its own conscious experience, but may know that of other individuals only indirectly, by its effects. Relative to one individual, the others could be considered "unconscious."

Cohesive Self

I use a formal definition of Cohesive Self abstracted from that of Kohut (1971) as "that which experiences itself as a mental and physical unit having extension in space and continuity in time." *The* Cohesive Self, with capital letters, refers to the sense of selfhood of a single human organism. With the exception of multiple personalities and fragmented schizophrenics, this is experienced as a unity. For myself, it is the experience of being John Beahrs, whatever it is that distinguishes that from the sum of my parts or any single part.

The theory of co-consciousness assumes that *each part* of any human individual has some sense of selfhood of its own, discrete from that of other parts and the Self proper, with "selfhood" defined nearly in the same way as above. With Self and selves being nearly the same in definition, and often very difficult to separate in actual point of fact, the definition of selfhood has already become fuzzy.

Unconscious

I use the term "unconscious," or *the* unconscious proper, in keeping with scientific convention and for clinical utility. It is the collective of all aspects or parts of an individual's mind of which the Cohesive Self proper is not aware, except through their effects. For myself, it is all aspects of myself which for John Beahrs are normally out of awareness. I use the term in both the psychoanalytic and hypnotic connotations, while preferring the latter, and discuss these in some depth in Chapter 4. But co-consciousness assumes that each part of this "unconscious" must have its own ongoing *conscious* experience. There can then be no such thing as an unconscious, in any absolute sense. "Unconscious" can only be relative to one particular part. For part-self A, for example, part-selves B, C, D, and E may all be beyond awareness. If A dominates the entire individual's Cohesive Selfhood, then the latter four would be part of *the* unconscious. But they are not asleep. Called forth, each could report its own identity, experience, and perspectives, which might differ dramatically from one another and from A. A might or might not be in its *own* "unconscious." If the Cohesive Self proper shifts control between different part-selves, what is unconscious would shift depending upon which part-self carried selfhood proper or was "out." The term "unconscious," a fiction in the most absolute sense, is already becoming blurry and confused—fuzzy. Yet clinical utility and its correspondence to common experience militate against totally abandoning the term.

The most central unresolved issue which all of this poses, raised in Chapters 4 and 6 but by no means resolved, is by what means one's sense of continuity of overall Selfhood proper becomes established, given a potentially infinite number of separate selves within. Looking upon an individual as like a symphony orchestra, how is the conductor set up and maintained in office? And in disturbed psychiatric patients where stable selfhood is lacking, what should be our priorities in determining who *should* wield the baton? The issue of *the* "conscious," when actually all parts are simultaneously conscious, probably resolves to this issue of the *executive*—which part(s) controls the body and can make itself known to other human individuals. That a human organism can go through an entire biological life span with many, if not most, part-selves never having this opportunity is certainly food for thought. And quite a large bite, at that.

The concept of simultaneous co-consciousness within a single human individual is what distinguishes the theoretical position of *Unity and Multiplicity* from the many psychiatric theories which talk about component parts of a personality. Here, parts are not abstractions or mechanisms, but consciously experiencing beings *with whom we can and must communicate*. It is upon this premise that almost all of my suggestions for clinical technique are predicated. To clarify how this premise itself is derived requires close scrutiny of the issues behind ambiguity, imprecision, and fuzzy thinking.

Logic of Co-consciousness

1) Hidden observers, with an independent sense of selfhood simultaneous with and distinct from that of the subject, are found to be present in hypnotized subjects. This is a demonstrable empirical datum, whatever conclusions we might attach to it.
2) Co-consciousness is the rule in normal hypnotic states (restatement of #1).
3) Hypnosis cannot be separated from non-hypnotic waking states without logical absurdity. They are simply polar opposite ways of experiencing and perceiving what in actuality is a unified continuum.
4) What is applicable to hypnosis must in some meaningful sense also be applicable to non-hypnotic waking states, and vice versa.
5) Hidden observers must be present in all non-hypnotic waking as well as in hypnotic experience (conclusion from premises #1 and #4). Hence, *co-consciousness must be present in all normal waking life*.

Granting the above logic, Hilgard's (1977) research on *the* "hidden observer" strongly suggests at least a dual consciousness, though not necessarily multiplicity. The duality might correspond fairly closely to the "conscious-unconscious" dichotomy as used by most hypnotists (cf. Chapter 4), whose therapeutic implications are best reviewed by LeCron (1964). The Self 1 and Self 2 concepts (Gallwey, 1974; Beahrs, 1977a, b) are equally relevant here. Additional research on hidden observers by Watkins and Watkins (1979a) provides the data from which we are led inexorably to a position of *multiple* co-consciousness inherent in our basic "unity."

6) Different hidden observers are found, empirically, when different hypnotic states are investigated in the same individual subject. These appear to have different personality styles of their own, prefer a different mode of address, and perform a different role in the overall personality organization or Self. Like premise #1, this is a replicable empirical datum from the research laboratory.

7) To avoid absurdity, we must be able to look on every different human experience as a different type of hypnotic state. This is a re-statement of premises #3 and #4.

8) As every human moment is different from every other, any human individual experiences an *infinite* number of different hypnotic states, infinite at least in the sense of there being no finite limit.

9) There can be an unlimited, potentially infinite number of hidden observers or "personalities" within a single human individual. *Unlimited co-consciousness* follows from premises #6 and #8.

Few scientists would have trouble with premises #1, #2, and #6 in the above. These represent data which are increasingly well accepted as reliable from the research laboratory. If premise #4 and its coro-lary premise #8 can be held with reasonable confidence, we can hold equally reasonable confidence in the conclusion: that multiple co-consciousness without a specific finite limit is the rule and not the exception in human experience. But *is* whatever is found out about hypnosis of equal relevance to non-hypnosis? And vice versa? Of what value, then, is our even defining the one condition as separate or different from the other?

The weak points in the logic seem clearly to fall into the rubric of premises #3, #4, #7 and #8 — that all experience can be considered as hypnotic. These reduce to a common denominator: that to separate non-hypnotic from hypnotic in any absolute sense involves both logi-cal and practical absurdity. Yet I stated at the very beginning of this book that much of the content material has come from years of exper-ience working with hypnosis. Of what relevance is a study of hypnosis — or study of anything, for that matter — unless it is something special? If existence of anything (A) can have meaning only if contrasted with that which is outside of its boundaries or domain (Not-A), of what relevance can this discussion be?

Fuzzy thinking dominates the picture, at least in this central and critical area. Why this *must* be so I hope to clarify in the next section. And it is here that the *type* of fuzzy thinking departs from what could otherwise simply be sloppy research or loose writing. From the basic underpinnings of this imprecision have been derived not only the necessity of the imprecision itself, but conclusions about the nature of our minds which have massive implications both for psychiatry and psychotherapy, and for our basic understanding of ourselves and our place in the natural order. And this conclusion is *testable*, and so remains clearly within the domain of science—that which can be measured and tested.

While fuzzy thinking may remain offensive to those who crave precision, it may have the paradoxical side effect of leading to conclusions which themselves can be tested. While "science" at one level appears to have been abandoned, its scope is actually expanded by that very same process. This has its parallel in physics, where for over a half century scientists have been forced to abandon totally precise understanding as impossible even in principle, and have found out to their joy that the limits of their science have been expanded rather than limited. Perhaps psychiatric theory is now ready to take the same plunge from 19th-century determinism into that initially frightening realm where ambiguity must be accepted as a fact of life, whose implications must be faced and dealt with, whether we like it or not.

PSYCHIC UNCERTAINTY

One psychoanalyst summarized his critique of my approach as follows: "Underneath my basically critical posture towards your work is a *fear* . . . I fear that were I to follow your train of thought to its ultimate conclusions, my thinking would necessarily become more and more fuzzy. I would no longer be able to conceptualize human problems of living in a scientifically precise manner. And it is very important to me — yes, essential — to be able to think clearly, with scientific precision." As I pondered these comments, I not only appreciated my critic's respectful candor, but reflected upon just how profound the implications of his concern are. His fears are not only well founded, but perhaps unavoidable. It is indeed possible that one cannot discuss the issues at hand in a scientifically precise manner without ending up in absurdity — *even in principle*. Perhaps, even, the more one attempts to become precise, the more absurd his conclusions become. The more one retains an optimal *im*precision, the more flexibility the theory or model retains. My critic was more assuaged by the comment that the approach seems to *work* in certain areas of clinical practice, specifically where established theory proves tedious and cumbersome at best. Even within scientific circles, it is hard to argue with results.

Within the domain of physics, this very same fear was carried to his deathbed by no less a figure than Albert Einstein. Whatever kind of precise natural order might ultimately withstand the rigors of scientific testing would be acceptable to him, he claimed, but he could not bring himself to accept the idea of uncertainty as fundamental to the very nature of natural substance. These ambiguities did not evaporate or disappear, however, in deference to either his feelings or his towering stature. Nor did the whole fabric of science crash in ruins. To the contrary, quantum uncertainty has played a major role in one of the greatest theoretical achievements of the 20th century, the unification of chemistry and physics into a single framework whose basic principles remain relatively simple. Again, it *worked,* and in physics also it is hard to argue with results.

I am increasingly convinced that imprecision or fuzzy thinking within the domain of *Unity and Multiplicity* is not merely an expression of my own unavoidable inadequacies, nor of the fact that my beliefs remain in a state of formulation and reformulation. I suspect that it reflects a fundamental principle of knowledge comparable in many ways to Heisenberg's Uncertainty Principle. It is not possible, even in principle, to have complete or precise knowledge of both the position and momentum of an elementary particle, even though precise knowledge of that particle would require both. The more we know of the location of the particle, the less we know what that particle is doing (direction of motion, velocity, etc.) and vice versa. Uncertainty (imprecision) is hence unavoidable, and can be formulated in relatively simple mathematical form, $\Delta x \Delta p_x \geq h/2\pi$, where Δx represents uncertainty of position, Δp_x uncertainty of momentum, and the complex of $h/2\pi$ is a numerical constant (Teller, 1980).

If there is little reason to fear imprecision in that most "precise" of all sciences, physics, there is even less within the psychological domain. Ambiguity, paradox, and tension between polar opposites have been recognized and accepted as essential features of the human condition since the time of the ancient Greeks. As with Einstein, even the most ardent desire for tightly precise "scientific" understanding will not automatically create this where it is necessarily lacking. And if uncertainty has expanded rather than limited the scope of physics, there is no a priori reason why this cannot also be the case in psychology and psychiatry. In these disciplines, as in physics, certain areas of inquiry push these limits more than others.

Those areas where psychic uncertainty seems to hold sway are specifically those which have defiantly escaped scientific consensus within all disciplines up to the present time. Examples are free will vs. determinism, hypnosis vs. non-hypnosis, good vs. evil, God vs. materialism, etc. These challenge and transgress the limits of relevance of every precise theory I have ever encountered. Yet they remain as essential to issues of mental health as they have been throughout all recorded history. Hence they cannot be ignored without terrible cost, and it behooves us at least to search out and identify the underpinnings of this imprecision. What emerges can then be further defined, clarified, elaborated upon, and tested from many different perspectives. The primarily clinical data discussed in this book are presented as content material to be subjected to this further scrutiny.

If it is possible to formulate a psychic uncertainty principle in even quasi-mathematical terms, this increases the likelihood that co-consciousness, and much of the blurred categories we encounter when working with it, will be given a fair hearing by the scientific community. Those who justly require clear and rigorous thinking will be more satisfied the more this type of thinking can clearly and rigorously demonstrate that blurring of boundaries may be more an asset than a liability. It will then be difficult to relegate such an important area of inquiry as multiple consciousness to the second-class realm of the "occult," to be discounted by most scientists as if it didn't exist, but all-too-eagerly swallowed up by the discontented fringes. I value scientific respectability too much, like my psychoanalytic critic, not to do my best to deserve and win such respect.

The closest I can come at present to a precise statement of why scientific precision is impossible, especially within the subject matter of this book, is what in Chapter 2 I have called the A/Not-A Absurdity. Mathematically, it seems like a fairly simple, commonsense boundary phenomenon. *If boundaries between A and Not-A are imprecise or blurred in actual point of fact, and yet to distinguish these categories from one another is necessary to denote an important dimension of human experience, it is not hard to intuit that the more precision is attempted, the less reliability, and vice versa.* And this paradox is especially applicable to the subject matter of *Unity and Multiplicity.* I will state the train of logic in its bare essentials, basically a repeat of the brief exposition in Chapter 2. I will then share several examples from the many areas of life and common experience where this principle must apply and hopefully show why this is more the case in some areas of inquiry than in others.

The A/Not-A Absurdity

1) Define A and Not-A in clear operational terms to which most people can relate, each denoting an experientially distinct dimension of life experience.
2) Collect objective data.
3) Logical analysis of #2, the data, in terms of #1, the original definitions themselves, leads to conclusions which violate the premises and/or the data.

What was formerly seen as A can now be seen as "really" Not-A, and vice versa, even though neither the facts nor the definitions have been changed. In either case, the definitions appear to lose relevance. This does violence to the fact that the original distinctions of A and Not-A, whether or not they logically hold up, referred to dimensions of human experience which *seem* different from one another, based on observations which led to our defining these distinctions in the first place. The more precision is attempted in separating A from Not-A, the more we end up in absurdity. That the areas where this applies are as significant as voluntary vs. involuntary, good vs. evil, God vs. non-God, and the psychiatric dimensions of hypnosis and dissociative disorder forbids our turning out backs on the problem as though it were a mere intellectual exercise.

Let's look at some of the features of the A/Not-A Absurdity. Where applicable,

1) A and Not-A are at opposite poles along a *continuum*, along which
   boundaries are *arbitrary*.
2) Despite the above, our *experience* of A and Not-A as profoundly
   different from one another and of great importance to life issues,
   requires that we use labels to denote or refer to these different
   dimensions of experience.

I can perhaps illustrate this by looking again at Figures 2a and 2b
(see p. 19). If all points on the graphs are intended to comprise the
scope of any one individual's conscious experience, the ease with
which we can reliably differentiate two types of consciousness, along
the coordinates of the graph, depends on the presence of some type of
boundary between these in actual point of fact. For Mr. 2a, consciousness exists in basically two clusters, even though there are still
many points in the grey area between. Defining one cluster as hypnotic, another as non-hypnotic, is likely to become problematic only a
small portion of the time, when his consciousness is at the grey area
between. For individual 2b there is no discontinuity between A and
Not-A. The "grey area" would have to encompass virtually the entire
graph. Yet the dimensions referred to, especially voluntary and involuntary, do not disappear just because they are in continuity.
Hence we must attempt to make a differentiation in our theories in a
situation where there is no actual discontinuity to which these can correspond reliably. Whenever intellectual precision is attempted where
corresponding boundaries in point of fact can only be arbitrary, it
leads to this absurdity.

Figure A-1 schematizes a realm of discourse, such as hypnosis and

Figure A-1

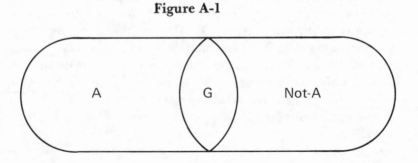

non-hypnosis, where we find it necessary to differentiate an A from a Not-A even though the two are just opposite poles along a continuum. G is defined as the *grey area* between A and Not-A. In a true continuum, the definition of G is also arbitrary, but has significant practical consequences which can be delineated. If *precision* (P) is defined as an attempt to define the sharpest possible boundary between A and Not-A, and *reliability (R)* as the degree to which our definitions of A and Not-A remain consistent and free of contradiction, we can then make several quasi-mathematical statements. Their meaning will hopefully become clearer with the real life examples which follow.

- The degree of A/Not-A Absurdity is inversely proportional to the size of G, the grey area permitted, and directly proprotional to P, or attempted precision.
- The more grey area is permitted (more G, less P), the more *reliability* will be inherent in our definitions (more R). The more precision, the less reliability.
- If precision is precisely defined as the reciprocal of the grey area G, I can formulate the *Psychic Uncertainty Principle* as follows:

$$R \alpha 1/P, \ P \alpha 1/R, \ \text{or} \ RP \alpha C, \text{where C is a constant.}$$

Comparing this to Heisenberg's Uncertainty Principle in physics, the variables of precision and reliability would correspond to those of position and momentum. The more precisely we know the one, the less we know the other. Precision is, and *must be*, limited. There are some differences. For one, the physical uncertainty principle was derived more from the interaction effects of the observer and the observed, the psychic one more from the necessity of defining distinctions where in reality the boundaries are blurred or only relative. The first element is also present in psychic uncertainty whenever measures cannot be clearly and unambiguously made, which is the case in all save the first of the examples which follow.

The constant C is a measure of how much precision can be permitted before reliability drops below whatever level is defined as acceptable. Within any one frame of reference, the value of C remains a numerical constant. This value is different in different settings, however. In Figure 2 (p. 19), common sense suggests that we can distinguish hypnosis from non-hypnosis with far greater reliability for Mr. 2a than for Mr. 2b. This is because the boundary can correspond to an actual area of separation between the two separate clusters of points of consciousness. Where no such boundaries actually exist, as in 2b, they can only be arbitrary. With physical objects, like a given chair, it is easy to define A separately from Not-A with nearly universal agreement.

This finds mathematical expression in the value of the constant C. The clearer the actual physical boundaries separating A from Not-A, the larger the value of C. For an object as discrete as a chair, the value of C is so high that reliability in defining the chair is not impaired until precision is attempted at a level approaching quantum uncertainty. But at this level the problem still emerges; no boundaries are absolute. Psychological and psychiatric theories deal with boundaries which, while not necessarily any less real, are much less discrete in point of fact. The value of C will here be low. Even small attempts at increasing precision, ones most scientists would accept as reasonable, may nonetheless result in a decrement in reliability which most of us would agree is *not* acceptable or "reasonable."

The *limits of relevance* of a construct, L, are the scope of this construct where reliability in our use of this construct remains within an acceptable range. The *domain* of the construct is the area enclosed within these limits. "Construct" refers to our concept of any organization of energy, and can refer to as different levels of abstraction as perception of objects (like the chair), definition of a concept relating to observable variables (like hypnosis), or even actual theoretical systems. Using Figure A-1, the limits of relevance of the definition of hypnosis refer to the area to the left of the grey area G. Since the size of the grey area permitted and the reliability required will vary from investigator to investigator, defining whether or not something is within or beyond the limits of relevance will be a judgment call, but it is still something for which guidelines could be suggested.

Because of the low values of C, limits of relevance of any specific psychiatric theory which attempts to be precise will be far less than those in the physical sciences. Even that which denotes our basic identity, what Kohut calls Cohesive Self, is felt to be defined by boundaries which are loose and constantly shifting. That something as precious as our own identity cannot be precisely and reliably defined may be threatening, but can bring home a humbling awareness of our own limits, and a willingness to think of ourselves in less absolute or either/ or manner than customary.

EXAMPLES

While psychic uncertainty in the hypnotic/non-hypnotic dimension is of the greatest relevance for this work, I will preface its discussion with two other examples intended to clarify and bring to life the practical as well as logical consequences of precision and imprecision. The first is taken from the poorly defined intersection between medicine and psychiatry. Since it involves measurable boundary definitions which can be rigidly adhered to, it illustrates the practical but not the logical aspect of the A/Not-A Absurdity. The second example — defining good and evil as the A and Not-A — is philosophical and hits at the core of our most basic life issues. Upon what do we found our basic values, an ethical structure necessary for cooperative social living? Here the interdependence of one upon the other pole renders precise definition of A as separate from Not-A impossible even in principle. This renders A/Not-A into a necessary absurdity at the logical level as well. This is a true example of the Psychic Uncertainty Principle applied to the domain of ethics.

A similar problem pervades defining hypnosis in relation to non-hypnosis. This is a paradigm of the free will vs. determinism controversy in the context most amenable to scientific and clinical study. What distinguishes voluntary vs. involuntary function has long been and remains one of the most significant unresolved issues in psychiatry. Co-consciousness emerges as a new concept from the very fact of why this dilemma is unresolvable. Paradoxically, it provides a new datum carrying the potential to resolve the paradox at another level.

Medical Examples
Hypoglycemia. Many clinicians have noted the extent to which some types of emotional hyperreactivity syndromes seem to parallel the disturbed glucose tolerance found in some pre-diabetics, alcoholics, post-gastrectomy patients and others. A common factor is a postprandial drop in blood sugar to well below the resting fasting level.

The persistently impaired frustration tolerance in these patients is sometimes thought to reflect a physiological readjustment of the stress-adrenalin response, which itself is an adaptation to frequent fluctuations in blood sugar. If more adrenalin is secreted per unit stress, this may manifest psychiatrically as less frustration tolerance, greater anxiety, and a worsening of any type of psychiatric symptoms to which a particular patient might be predisposed. Many of these patients will show a dramatic improvement in stress tolerance or "ego strength" when simply placed on a hypoglycemic diet structured to keep the blood sugar levels as stable as possible. This is not a theoretical position, but an observation which needs explanation. The question is, do these patients *have* "hypoglycemia," implying a medical condition or illness for which a specific medical treatment is palliative if not curative?

Hypoglycemia differs from many other subjects within psychosomatic medicine in the extreme to which polarized views are held at either end of the A/Not-A continuum. There are believers and non-believers. One can be "for" hypoglycemia or "against" it; in either case, the position is hardly scientific. These positions can even be taken by otherwise scientifically sophisticated individuals.

In an attempt to solve this dilemma, most internists attempt a precise definition of hypoglycemia. Part of the currently accepted criteria is that to qualify for the diagnosis of hypoglycemia, the blood sugar must drop to or below 50 mg %, and this drop must be accompanied by mental symptoms.

Patient A presents with a classic emotional hyperreactivity syndrome and a drop in blood sugar to 49 mg% three hours postprandial confirms the diagnosis of hypoglycemia. This diagnosis is ratified by a dramatic improvement in emotional stress tolerance in response to a hypoglycemic diet. Patient B, however, presents an identical clinical picture, but his blood glucose drops to a minimum of 51 mg%, and the diagnosis is ruled out. But 49 and 51 are so close as to approach identity in actual value, and patient B is nearly as likely as A to respond to the same treatment. But since he does not have hypoglycemia, treatment as such might be deferred. Hence the absurdity.

Many clinicians have noted a dramatic response to hypoglycemic diet by many patients whose glucose tolerance is far less disturbed than the "real" hypoglycemia described above. Since clinical results are what count, they argue that perhaps the criteria for hypoglycemia should be loosened. With less stringent criteria for the diagnosis, the "disease" then becomes very common, afflicting nearly the majority of human adults. They approach an "everything is A" position which seems absurd to most practicing physicians. I should note that simply raising the cutoff point would not solve the dilemma. More hypoglycemics would be diagnosed, and fewer non-hypoglycemics, but if 60 mg% were the new precise criterion, we would still have the same dilemma that two virtually identical patients would be defined and treated differently, Mrs. C with 59 and Mr. D with 61. Wherever we draw the line, the problem is the same — attempts at overprecision where such is lacking in point of fact.

Some physicians have noted that many psychiatrically healthy individuals will show disturbed glucose tolerance, with drop in sugar levels into the 40's or even 30's, with few if any mental symptoms or need for special diets. They then will take a nearly "everything is Not-A" position. If the criterion is made more strict, however, the dilemma persists.

Both of the groups, the A and the Not-A proponents, are correct as far as they go, but both neglect the importance of a grey area in between. Suppose that we deliberately sacrifice precision. We might define a person as having hypoglycemia if he is symptomatic and has a blood sugar drop below 40 mg%. We might say it is definitely *not* present if a person is asymptomatic and has a blood sugar remaining over 60 mg%. The area between would be a grey area or transitional zone, within which patients could not be judged according to the "rules" of hypoglycemia. They might be the fortunate recipients of more individualized assessment and treatment.

While there would still be occasional patients violating the principles of the definitions, these would be few. My guess is that now the vast majority of diagnoses of hypoglycemia would be appropriate, as would be those cases in whom the diagnosis is clearly ruled out. Deliberately sacrificing precision or increasing the grey area or transition zone, then, enhances the reliability of the concept of hypoglycemia by orders of magnitude, in cases where the criteria for A or Not-A are still met. The grey area simply acknowledges what in any case remains as a fact of life, that things are not always as clear-cut as we might like.

Example from Ethics

Good vs. Evil. All attempts throughout history to define an absolute system of ethical values have been thwarted by one simple but annoyingly incorrigible fact of life. If, even in principle, all members of a society were to agree on basic ethical premises, like the Ten Commandments, the problem would remain. Absolute, agreed-upon moral tenets unavoidably come into conflict with other absolute, agreed-upon tenets, within the arena of actual living. Whatever choices we make, we cannot avoid doing something which violates some "absolute." War is openly destructive and unloving—in a word, evil. But to roll over and submit to a Hitlerian tyranny is no less evil. So what do we do?

Attempts within the Catholic Church to define inviolable absolutes frequently challenge this absurdity in everyday life. Abortion and birth control, seen as anti-life, are conceived as *always* evil. Yet willful overextension of a parent's resources to the point that he cannot provide for even the basic needs of his offspring is also evil. Rigid adherence to the first may result in violation of the second absolute, the obligation of parents to do all they can to give their children a good start in the arena of life. But a staunch Catholic will argue that free sexual expression and abortion for convenience have not done wonders for the stability of our social structure. So perhaps abstinence is an answer. But willfully stifling the free expression of love within the marital union also weakens that union and itself threatens that social structure. The more rigidly one takes a stand at any point, the more doggedly the converse issues return to reduce the original stand to absurdity. Most interesting is that nearly opposite positions might be taken on social issues, such as "Right to Life," by individuals who would agree on all of the premises above. The difference arises from disagreement over priorities. If one value must go, which should go first?

I addressed this issue clearly in *That Which Is* (1977a), reaching the conclusion that judgments on good and evil by their very nature depend on what person or society is used as a reference point. Even using my suggestion of the "Society of Mankind" as a more absolute standard of reference will not resolve the clashes of value when applied to real life situations. Either/or boundaries between good and evil cannot be established *even in principle* for two reasons: 1) What is good from one reference point is evil from another, at the level of everyday life; 2) even from the same reference point, the same situation or event can usually be looked upon from either a positive or negative perspective, hence some of each polarity, with equal accuracy. While this may increase our flexibility and power for action, it hardly enhances our confidence in our moral absolutes. Is there little alternative to the chaos of total moral relativism??

Brill (1979) suggests an alternative. This is the concept of *moral presumption*. Recognizing the necessity of taking a strong moral stand in order to stabilize and organize social living, moral presumption suggests a way of establishing priorities. "Presumption" is used in exactly the same sense as in law, as in the presumption of "innocent until proven guilty." *The burden of proof* is upon he who would violate a basic ethical tenet. To embark upon some intrinsically evil venture, such as war, would require comparably stringent criteria as proof of guilt in a court of law — here, proof that beyond a reasonable doubt a worse evil would follow by not commiting the first evil. When faced with a Hitler, war may not only be less evil, but can even be the ''more loving'' course of action. But it is not to be taken lightly. It does (or at least should) require that burden of proof.

Burden of proof is a far more strict and difficult cirterion to satisfy than that whim of convenience which absolutists appropriately fear. While it might actually have resulted in America's entry into the Second World War sooner, when we became aware of the magnitude of the Holocaust and of Great Britain's peril of annihilation, other wars might have failed to pass this test.

Such a position does not weaken values in the slightest. Similar to the suggestion of deliberately allowing a grey area between the diagnoses of hypoglycemia and non-hypoglycemia, it enhances the reliability and hence the strength of such judgments once they are made. Fewer wars will be fought, as fewer diagnoses of hypoglycemia will be made, but those we do enter will be on a far more solid moral basis. Again, *deliberate loosening* of precision leads to *enhanced strength* and reliability of our judgments, when they are in fact made, outside the grey area. The grey area simply recognizes and acknowledges what will remain a fact of life whether we like it or not, that whatever bible we use, judgments must often be made on a case by case basis, and that strong opinions will necessarily differ.

Hypnosis and Non-Hypnosis

The three-factor definition of hypnosis which I suggested in Chapter 2 is intended to fit common usage as much as possible. Along each of three continua, "hypnosis" refers to a dimension of human experience distinctly different from non-hypnosis, although where we draw the boundary between one and the other must remain arbitrary. I will discuss the issue from the perspective of the *volitional* continuum. Not only is this as representative as the others, but also what distinguishes a freely chosen or "voluntary" act from one which "just happens" — with the vast social implications of *responsibility* — remains one of the most critical dilemmas in psychiatry (Beahrs, 1977a).

How the psychic uncertainty principle arises and applies to the domain of hypnosis is not unlike the prior two examples, especially the latter. Barber (1972) has repeatedly emphasized the Not-A position. His research has been set up to demonstrate the frequency with which effects most would agree are "hypnotic" arise equally significantly within a context most of us would call non-hypnotic. In place of customary hypnotic procedures, Barber uses a control of *task motivation*. Devoting maximal *conscious, volitional* energy towards the task at hand is at the extreme *non*-hypnotic end of the continuum. If this leads to paradoxical increase in experiences and behaviors which seem to "just happen," it becomes increasingly difficult to call these "hypnotic," if this word is intended to imply something uniquely distinct from the normal waking continuum.

The classic example is creating an experience of hypnotic arm rigidity not by "suggestion" but by free choice. Example: "Purposely extend your right arm and tighten all the muscles to the point that your arm feels *like* a rigid bar of iron that would be difficult to bend no matter how hard you tried. Tighten all of the opposing muscle groups to the point that your arm is fixed tightly in its extended position. Then choose to imagine your arm as if it were such an iron bar. *While doing both of the above*, try as hard as you can to bend your rigid arm but find that you cannot bend it no matter how hard you try." Many subjects will at least fleetingly experience that they *really can't* bend their arm no matter how hard they try. This is a hypnotic response which now seems involuntary. Yet that it is chosen is obvious, which violates the same criterion by which the response is judged as hypnotic.

Barber claims that all involuntary experience is basically similar in kind. It is clearly done by the subject (nobody else did it for him), but the *experience of awareness of the choice slips out of awareness* (sic). Dissociation reappears. What otherwise seems like a mind-game assumes life and death significance every time the insanity "defense" is raised in a court of law.

The polar opposite paradox is illustrated by a subject carrying out a *posthypnotic suggestion*. Example: A deeply hypnotized subject is given the suggestion that at some time long after he "awakens" he will hear three taps of the hypnotist's pen and, without any recall that the suggestion was given, he will then walk up to a bookshelf, pick out an arbitrarily chosen book, and throw it to the floor. Later in the evening, the subject indeed gets up from the group, walks over to the book-shelf, picks out a book, and dashes it to the floor. Someone asks him why he did such a seemingly foolish act. Rarely does he say that it was because he was given hypnotic suggestion. Sometimes he may reply, embarrassed, "I don't know what seemed to get into me." More often, however, he will give a "rational" explanation for his actions indistin-guishable to himself or others from one which might have been given for a similar action done outside of the hypnotic setting. He will give reasons why he *"chose"* his action which have little if any connection to hypnotic setting. The group will realize that his response "just hap-pened," but the subject experiences it as voluntary. If the process was both experientially and behaviorally the same as that of doing any "free act," is it not then more likely that all really free acts are also "really" determined, possibly by other events in a person's life which act as hypnotic suggestions? Everything is now seen as A (hypnotic).

It is not hard to see each of the above examples as a special case of the free will vs. determinism controversy as it applies to everyday life. What is chosen at one level just happens at another, and vice versa. The boundaries blur. For this if no other reason, to precisely separate hypnotic from non-hypnotic will lead to logical absurdity. That events can, like good and evil, be simultaneously A and Not-A renders precise boundary definitions impossible even in principle. As with ethics and hypoglycemia, the more we define a grey area between A and Not-A, the more our use of the terms will be reliable, free of contradictions. But this separation will never be absolute. And where we define the grey area is equally arbitrary, and subject to the same absurdities. In an absolute sense, then, hypnotic and non-hypnotic are truly inseparable, and what applies to one must apply to the other. As seen earlier, co-consciousness must follow as a corollary.

Similar thinking clouds current theoretical positions within the scope of the larger issue of freedom and responsibility, as opposed to determinism. To avoid contradiction between theory and data, many theorists are increasingly led to the polar A and Not-A positions. Freud and the early psychoanalysts assumed that all chosen acts were "really" determined, using logic similar to the case of the posthypnotic suggestion above, and subsequently ratified by its impressive explanatory value. But Roberts (1974) and many humanistic psychologists, supported by data similar to that of Barber, argue impressively that everything, *even physical reality*, is "freely chosen." This premise, which so violates our common sense perception of matter, is even given support by such physicists as Bohr (1961) and Teller (1980), who note how much the unpredictable behavior of elementary particles resembles and parallels that of human beings. As I had suggested in *That Which Is*, this emphasizes that if everything is made of the same "stuff," this may be in essence more like our "minds" than like the everyday perception of "matter."

The polar opposite "all A" and "all Not-A" positions presented above actually have more in common than not. Both discount the *experiential* distinction between voluntary and involuntary actions, which demands to be dealt with in everyday life whether or not the distinction is absurd! Common experience, which also does not go away in deference to anyone's feelings or stature, demands that we make distinctions which, carried to their logical conclusions, become absurd.

Co-consciousness emerges as a conclusion from our inability to meaningfully separate hypnosis from the waking state in general, as already shown. If/when validated by scientific experiment and clinical utility, the logic can also proceed in an opposite direction. If co-consciousness is now taken as an experimentally demonstrable datum occurring throughout all waking experience, this will strengthen the position that psychic uncertainty is a principle which cannot be violated without logical as well as practical absurdity. If status along the dichotomies of voluntary-involuntary and conscious-unconscious can be defined only relative to which coexisting ego state is taken as a reference point, it would be impossible even in principle to define any boundary between poles of these dichotomies for any larger aggregate of consciousness such as a Cohesive Self. With psychic uncertainty further demonstrable, co-consciousness is increasingly validated. Paradoxes resolve at another level. And hypothesis becomes scientific theory, from which many predictions can be made which are amenable to scientific testing.

Appendix II:

The Hillside Strangler:

Mad, Bad, or Multiple?

When Kenneth Bianchi was apprehended by authorities as the prime suspect for a series of brutal rape-murders attributed to the "Hillside Strangler," he appeared perplexed. He had never been in serious trouble with the law and had proven himself capable not only of gainful employment but of at least adequate functioning in the roles of husband and father. With women he was respectful in his feelings, attitudes, and behaviors — perhaps a bit on the meek and mild-mannered side. He reported no recall or awareness of anything even peripherally related to the grisly deeds for which he was charged, and that he could be a murderously sadistic rapist and cold-blooded killer seemed as foreign to his character as night from day.

Two disquieting features persisted, however. First, he readily acknowledged that with increasing frequency in his adult life there were periods of time which he lost track of — amnesic episodes, "blackouts" or whatever — which to him were as if they did not even exist. While he had to that point not had any evidence that these were a serious problem, they had certainly given him reason to stop and think — to wonder about what was going on. Worse, the evidence brought to bear against him by the criminal investigators was so thorough and conclusive that there could be no question even in his own mind that he was, in fact, that notorious Hillside Strangler. At least it could be proven that his body raped and then murdered the victims. But who was the "he" who was guilty? Ken Bianchi claimed no awareness of the heinous offenses which appeared so demonstrably out of character for him. Could there be *another* "he" within Ken's body? Or even more? If so, could Ken be truly responsible and culpable for his offenses, as required by law before criminal penalties can be meted out? If not Ken, then who?

Three facts of the case are sufficiently established that they will be stated, and used as assumptions upon which the remainder of this discussion will be based. First, there is no question of Kenneth Bianchi's guilt. The evidence shows that, without any reasonable doubt, he or at least his body caused the sexual violation and death of many female victims. Secondly, his life history seemed totally incongruous with such atrocities. Third, he claimed no awareness of anything even resembling the criminal offenses themselves or the type of impulses which one would expect to underlie these. And he seemed fairly convincing in his presentation.

The primary issue, both legal and psychiatric, brought before the court was to decide between two possible explanations, which were seen by nearly all concerned to be polar opposite, contradictory, and irreconcilable — at least in their legal implications. First, is Bianchi a multiple personality? If his offenses were committed in a dissociated state over which Ken had not even a glimmer of awareness, let alone control, then how could he even remotely have known the nature and consequences of his actions sufficiently to warrant criminal responsibility? In other words, is he "not guilty by reason of insanity"? *Or* were the offenses "instrumental acts," committed by a conscious choice of the entire organism, with claims of amnesia being a deliberate lie used as a smoke screen to obscure his culpability and escape the consequences? If so, he is a psychopath who is not only responsible for his actions, but should pay the highest penalty — both for protection of society and as a deterrent to other potential offenders. The question boiled down to the differential diagnosis of multiple personality or antisocial personality. Mad or bad?

I am presenting this case, now a part of the public record, as a separate appendix as an example *par excellence* not only of differential

diagnostic dilemmas in dissociative disorder, but of many other ramifications of *Unity and Multiplicity* as well. These are legal, moral,
logical, scientific, philosophical, and psychiatric. Psychic uncertainty
or the A/Not-A Absurdity rears its ugly head at several levels to such a
degree that it cannot be dismissed. First and foremost is the free will-
determinism controversy as blatantly as it can be found in its everyday
life context. To determine precisely whether an action was freely
chosen or involuntarily "just happened" becomes absurd in this case,
even though the consequences of this determination are of life and
death significance for the accused. The internal and external flaws in
the "insanity defense" demonstrate the legal manifestation of this absurdity.

Secondly, the case illustrates the absurdities to which rigid either-
or positions in psychiatry can lead, which sometimes become embar-
rassing to our profession when exposed in a court of law. This case was
especially striking for the extent to which such noted experts in psychiatry and hypnosis as J. G. Watkins and M. T. Orne reached polar
opposite positions, despite having done exhaustive in-depth evaluations of the case, using their expertise as well as the full body of objective information available. Not only could neither be budged from his
position but, with as objective an outside assessment as I am capable,
I can find no basis upon which either party should necessarily be forced
to budge. As different as their positions are, each may be true, at least
at one level — or, true but only part of the story.

Another set of issues exemplified by this case is related to the extent
to which the evaluating experts' preliminary bias can and perhaps
must influence the course and outcome of the evaluation, no matter
how hard they try to be objective. Once they arrive at a tentative position, do they selectively elicit information supporting this position
and selectively exclude that which might lead them to consider viable
alternatives? If the subject of the examination behaves differently
with each examiner, in a way supportive of the examiner's expectations and/or covert wishes, does that mean he is is "playing the
system" and is at least covertly dishonest or openly sociopathic? Or
does this also reflect what is again an unavoidable fact of life within
psychiatry? An examiner must formulate certain presuppositions in
order to structure and direct further inquiries, and his or her behavior
will of course vary depending upon the nature of these presupposi-

tions. And no human being can avoid responding differently to interviewers whose implied positions, communicated at so many covert as well as overt levels, are different. When neither positions wilts away even when *all* the data are subjected to the objectifying scrutiny of a court of law, I prefer to step away from such tempting and facile pseudo-explanations as narrowmindedness and ill will, and examine the possibility that something much more profound is being illustrated. More than one thing can be occurring, at many levels and at all times.

Does what best explains the data necessarily lead to the most desirable pragmatic outcome? One could argue, in the Bianchi case, that the diagnosis of multiple personality is more appropriate clinically than that of antisocial personality, and yet also argue that the most desirable disposition is a finding of "guilty" and a sentence of life imprisonment without possibility of parole. If this were the case, the integrity of everyone concerned would be pushed. Would we fudge on diagnostic accuracy in order to facilitate a most desirable outcome, the protection of society? Or would we remain true to our scientific integrity, even knowing that the outcome could be unfortunate or even tragic to innocent victims? Or, perhaps, when this dilemma occurs in such blatant form, we would do well to re-examine the relationships we have defined between beliefs and actions. This could be at the level of diagnosis and disposition, which in this particular case would involve the entire reexamination of the criminal insanity concept. At another level, it involves a reexamination of the relationship between psychiatric theory and the technical psychiatric behaviors we believe to be linked to the theory. By what means are the two linked? Are there desirable alternatives?

I will start with the evidence supporting a clinical diagnosis of multiple personality, doing this for two reasons. First, while I am arguing that the differential in this particular case is more either-and than either-or, I still believe that multiple personality is more appropriate clinically. Secondly, multiplicity is the primary emphasis of this book, and the case is an excellent illustration of problems we encounter in diagnosis. Here are the case highlights as they emerged through the evaluation by J. G. Watkins:

(a) The life history was incompatible with a diagnosis of antisocial personality. Not only did he *not* have a history of delinquent behavior prior to age 15, a necessary criterion for the antisocial, but his record was also entirely clean, until the present. Furthermore, he had proven himself capable of sustained employment, and functioned adequately in the role of husband and father. These also violate the criteria for a diagnosis of antisocial personality. If this were his diagnosis — simple "bad guy" — he would be atypical to say the least. Nor is he or was he psychotic in any blatant form. Clearly, something else must be going on. A history of an increasing problem with amnesic episodes or "blackouts" suggests that we at least take a look at major dissociative disorder.

(b) The accused agreed to undergo formal hypnosis, but proved to be quite resistant initially — this is not typical of multiple personalities except when fearful of what might be disclosed. Several tests were given to satisfy the examiner that the hypnotic state was for real — not simulated or malingered.

(c) "Perhaps there is some part of Ken with whom I have not yet talked. If there is, let the right hand lift." This statement-suggestion was intended to elicit any dissociated part-personality which might be present, with neither its existence or characteristics being necessarily defined. The right hand lifted. This hypnotic hand levitation was a signal from an aspect of the personality with whom the investigator had not yet talked. "Would that part come out and communicate with me?" There was considerable delay, but finally a dramatic personality change.

The patient now called himself "Steve" and ventilated his hatred of many people, especially Ken. "I really fixed that turkey up good," describing how smart he was, how dumb Ken was, and how he deliberately set up the crimes so that Ken would be apprehended and pay the price. In prison, Steve reported, Ken would be weakened so much further that he (Steve) would be able to fully take over the body. The crimes were gloatingly described in all their grisly detail, with not the slightest trace of guilt or remorse. In fact, while Ken had been satisfactorily married, Steve could be potent only with a female he intended to murder. The personality change could hardly have been more dramatic, as Watkins described in his report:

> Mildness changed to violence; reticence to talk about the crimes changed to bragging about them; soft voice changed to shout-

ing; respectful words in talking about women changed to crude obscenities; posture and gestures were different; good use of the English language changed to short ignorant verbalisms; solid, cognitive reasoning now became concrete, childish exclamations. The personality changed in all modalities, perceptual, intellectual, emotional, and motor.

Such a dramatic and sudden personality change is characteristic of multiple personality, which so often represents a tension between near opposites. What distinguishes a "for real" multiple from a malingerer is the consistency in one particular personality state over time in all modes, contrasted with the equally consistent but different behavior of the other personality states.

(d) Steve was aware of all that Ken said and did, but detailed inquiry failed to reveal any awareness of Steve's existence on the part of Ken. All the latter knew of Steve was the amnesic episodes. This is the classic one-way amnesic barrier, present to a variable degree in many multiples. Steve confirmed that he had concealed his presence from Ken, and ordered the examiner not to change that state of affairs. When Ken was reactivated, he claimed to have total amnesia for Steve. The evaluator did suggest, however, that "in your own way, at your own speed, you'll find out about Steve — you'll get stronger and stronger and Steve will be weaker and weaker." This is not an undesirable goal for therapy, to be sure, but was unfortunate for subsequent forensic evaluations where a major diagnostic criterion would be the permeability or impermeability of the ego state boundaries, and their consistency across different investigators.

(e) The life history which emerged seemed not only discordant with antisocial personality, but classic for the most severely disturbed type of dissociative disorder. Three key elements in Bianchi's childhood environment maximized not only the likelihood of dissociation, if he possessed that skill to begin with, but the malevolence of that dissociated entity. First, his mother was described as sadistically punitive, often doing such things as holding the boy's hand over a lighted flame to the point of agonizing pain, with little or no provocation. Secondly, expression of anger was forbidden, itself resulting in harsh sadistic retribution. Third, the mother was reportedly sexually seductive with the boy.

Experience of rage was not only likely in such an environment, but fueled with extra fire by an indelible association to the sexual drive. Yet its expression was forbidden. Such a vital part of that child's basic being would hardly go away by wishing it away. Ken did what is common in a creative latency-aged individual; he created an imaginary playmate whom he called "Steve." Initially no more than that, just an imaginary playmate created to provide solace, this construct provided a release from the pressure cooker. If the intolerable but still inexpressible sex-tinted rage could be attributed to, or projected into, this entity, it would feel less oppressive. Eventually this entity was disowned, and what first occurred with the child's full conscious awareness slipped beyond awareness and hence beyond voluntary control. However, it did not disappear. Ken might feel more comfortable, and even lead a marginally satisfactory life, but Steve would always be there, whether or not "out," carrying much of Ken's vital life energy. As a recipient for disowned rage, Steve was a classic *avenger*, an avenger who would "avenge" against innocent victims who only symbolically represented the original hate object.

The part-selves' attitude toward their mother was classic for this type of dissociation. Ken, who had "succeeded" in dealing with his rage by disowning it into Steve, reported good feelings about "*my* mother," and did not even like others to criticize her. Steve, however, reported that "I hate *his* (Ken's) mother". Here is the subject-object split, which comes up again and again at so many levels in these people. Ken had disowned Steve, for reasons which seemed obvious enough. Steve, for equally obvious reasons, not only disliked the mother, but developed increasing hatred for Ken himself, who had created Steve and subjected him to the double abuse of having to carry the burden of rage which Ken couldn't or wouldn't accept, and of being kept under a lid.

Much was made of Ken's half-hearted and futile attempts to become a policeman and psychologist, during the forensic dispute. He had achieved a deputyship in a police department, had dabbled with reading in psychology, and reportedly had fleeting contact with a lay hypnotist. Were these part of a long and carefully planned nefarious scheme that sometime in the future he would commit some senseless crimes and skillfully hide his guilt by feigning mental disorder? Or would as weak and insecure a part-personality as Ken perhaps be attracted to police work to get some sense of the power which he lacked, and to psychology for the comparable self awareness he so desperately needed?

During high school, a time with no overt personality changing, Ken did a piece of sculpture of a two-faced head. On the front was a normal human face, on the back a monster. With that uncanny wisdom of artistic creativity, this was a true and accurate portrayal of what the artist himself was not aware of in his usual conscious executive state.

(f) Psychological testing was done, both to clarify the diagnostic picture as much as possible and to ensure its validity. Watkins administered several tests, to both Ken and Steve, most notably the Rorshach. Ken was cooperative; Steve required much cajoling, but nonetheless did complete the tests. Separately, as if they were truly done by separate human individuals, they were submitted without identifying information to two of the most highly qualified experts for evaluation and interpretation. Ken was described by the evaluators as near-normal — perhaps mildly neurotic, introverted, having adequate reality testing, and normal ego centrality. Steve, on the other hand, was described as "one of the sickest I've seen." Violent sexual-aggressive impulses against women were found. The psychologists predicted that he probably was or would be a violent rapist and killer, and could be safe only in a high security state institution. He was described as possibly psychopathic, possibly covertly schizophrenic; more evidence was felt to be needed.

Of greatest significance for multiplicity is that both profiles were internally consistent. In a psychological test administered separately to different ego states or alter-personalities, strikingly different profiles, each with adequate validity scales indicating honesty and internal consistency, would suggest major dissociation. Poor validity scales could indicate faking or malingering, or simple defensiveness. Or, if the patient showed other indices of being genuine but validity scales were still off, it might reflect diffusion of ego state boundaries. Contamination of the responses of one ego state by those of another might reflect progress towards integration. Perhaps as dissociation is taken more seriously by the mental health profession, more sophisticated psychological tests will be developed to assess these and other possibilities.

In any case, Ken and Steve showed dramatically different profiles,

comparable to the two personalities' manifest behavior, and the validity gave at least presumptive evidence that they were "for real."
This is also a more formal way of stating the clinical impressions that
the case was so characteristic, and portrayed so convincingly, that for
it to have been willfully faked would have required acting ability,
knowledge of psychiatry, and basic intelligence far more extensive
than what the accused showed.

A third personality was subsequently uncovered with further hypnotic work. Going by the name of "Billy," this part-self had engaged
in some petty theft, and was also not known to the primary personality, Ken. I have little knowledge about Billy, his dynamics, etiology,
or role in the murder case. I understand that Ken himself had occasionally lied, in the sense known as "confabulation," when confronted
with behavior done during amnesic episodes of which he had no
awareness. I will make no attempt at a more exhaustive review, hoping that the material presented so far, along with the arguments for
sociopathy and the subsequent overview of the issues which follow,
will be sufficient for what is relevant to the reader of this book.

Watkins summarizes the argument for multiplicity tersely in his report, after quoting another evaluating expert's claim that no single
psychiatric diagnosis could possibly fit all the complexities and seeming contradictions involved.

> On the one hand he is a violent sexual deviate; on the other, a
> normal sexual individual; on the one hand, he is aggressive and
> murderous toward women; on the other, a loving husband and
> father; on the one hand, he hates his mother; on the other, he
> loves his mother; on the one hand he is passive; on the other he is
> violently active; on the one hand he seeks to be a policeman; on
> the other he steals — and when he steals he often returns what he
> has just stolen. Only in the context of different and separate per-
> sonalities, dissociated from one another and carrying out con-
> tradictory behaviors, can this make any sense.

Even if we were to assume that we now have nearly conclusive evidence that the accused is in fact a *bona fide* multiple personality, and
that the crimes were done in a dissociated state over which the primary personality had little, if any, control or even awareness, one

troublesome question remains. Now that the heinous deeds have been done, and we have established the accused's dangerousness to society whatever the diagnosis, what do we *do* with him? Is he "not guilty by reason of insanity"? As with clinical diagnosis, the expert witnesses were divided as to his legal sanity—a separate issue. While Watkins argued that Bianchi was a multiple personality, and that he was also legally insane, his recommendations hardly varied from those of the prosecution. The accused was extremely dangerous to others, a menace, and the likelihood of successful treatment was not secure enough to warrant the unconscionable risk to society of ever having him again on the loose. Recommendation: life imprisonment without possibility of parole, preferably in a high security mental ward rather than prison, but imprisonment nonetheless, for preservation of others. But this disposition is not compatible with a verdict of not guilty by reason of insanity. Here is the rub, and here, I believe, is why the prosecution invariably argues so vehemently against the diagnosis of multiple personality, and the court so often agrees. Perhaps if guilt and diagnosis were separate issues, as they should be at least logically, then forensic psychiatric diagnosis would be less contentious. This would require reexamination of the entire legal insanity concept.

Whether or not the legal insanity plea should be abolished in its current form, as I will argue later, that has not yet occurred. With the current statutes, a man such as the accused will be safely removed from society only if found guilty and sentenced to prison. This outcome is much more likely if the psychiatric diagnosis is one of sociopathy or antisocial personality, rather than multiple personality. This position was taken by M. T. Orne, himself one of the leading authorities on hypnosis and its place in psychiatry. And the arguments for that position are by no means trivial. I will now do my best to summarize the rather impressive evidence brought to bear against Bianchi, evidence which supports an alternative and seemingly exclusive diagnosis of antisocial personality, that he is more a simple evildoer than a true multiple.

The argument for the antisocial personality diagnosis follows:

(a) For an offense of this magnitude, with no question as to his actual guilt, a likely possibility not to be ruled out is that it is an *instrumental act*—i.e., one that is freely chosen, for which the subject is fully responsible. "I don't remember" is a common statement made by defendants, and the question is, what does the claim of amnesia mean? With criminal punishment at stake, it is not necessarily honest.

(b) The history is not entirely incompatible with antisocial personality. There is no police record, to be sure, but that may be the case only because charges were never filed. Deviancy of an antisocial type could conceivably be shown in the clinics rather than the courts, depending on how the behavior was expressed. Indeed, psychological records do show evidence of problems with school authorities, pimping for teenage runaways, and attempts at blackmail and extortion— all dealt with in the mental health instead of criminal justice system.

(c) Patient posed for a while as a sham psychologist, having temporarily convinced another psychologist that he was for real. To do this not only shows an individual quite capable of willful deception, but also gives evidence of the high intelligence and acting ability needed to convincingly feign or simulate such complex behaviors as hypnosis and multiple personality. When it becomes a matter of life or death, he would use this skill and knowledge to the utmost. There was also evidence that he had done at least a cursory study of hypnosis.

(d) There is considerable evidence that Ken was indeed simulating hypnosis. Orne, perhaps the leading authority on simulated hypnosis, put the accused through several of the tests which he himself had developed (Orne, 1959). These were tests of "trance logic" similar in nature to the example I used in Chapter 2: Given a suggestion for a negative hallucination, a simulating subject will bump into the individual whom he believes he shouldn't see, whereas the really hypnotized subject unobtrusively walks around the person he *really* doesn't see (but must see at some other level). In most cases the behavior of the accused showed to Orne what he would expect from a simulator, not the strange type of trance logic one finds in truly hypnotized subjects.

If one can successfully feign hypnosis, there is no particular reason why he could not do likewise with dissociative disorder. My own claim that the latter is a complicated version of the former, occurring spontaneously but beyond control, would certainly support this contention. In addition, Orne felt that he had proven at least one instance where the accused had deliberately lied to the investigator. When asked what the experience of hypnosis was like, the accused replied that it was "strange—like a light nap—seemed like a few minutes seemed like a few hours." Spontaneous time expansion is certainly an excellent indication of light hypnosis when there is no reason to suspect dishonest reporting, but it doesn't take too much knowledge to say the right thing to that question. Also, multiple personality is like spontaneous hypnosis at one level. If a subject is in hypnosis through much of his life, as one would expect for a true multiple, he would be less likely to report it as "strange." He would be much more likely to report it as similar to much of everyday living.

(e) The part-selves, Ken and Steve, had a "caricatured quality." Ken was just too good, Steve just too bad. Orne confronted Ken with the implausibility of his being such a "plastic saint," and then predicted that his behavior with the next interviewer would be less either-or. This was taken as further evidence that the accused was doing what he felt would most impress the interviewers.

(f) The accused is clearly behaving in a psychopathic manner, and is an antisocial personality even though quite atypical. He is guilty of the most reprehensible offenses, is an extreme danger to others, and should be dealt with accordingly by the law.

Seven expert witnesses in all were involved with the case. Opinions were divided on diagnosis, with a majority favoring that of dissociative disorder or multiple personality. There was also disagreement on whether or not he was legally insane. After repeated psychiatric examination and hypnosis sessions, the accused himself became convinced that he had done the killings. On the condition that the death penalty be dropped in return for his testimony against his accomplice, he confessed and pleaded guilty. He initially refused to let his attorney use the insanity defense, even though several evaluations supported this. Now in prison, his behavior is increasingly erratic — all of which can admit of more than one explanation.

DISCUSSION

Either-and

As I write out and then review my own abstract of the polar positions, multiplicity and antisocial personality, I find myself as nearly swayed by each position as if I were hearing it competently and eloquently argued in the courtroom. Studying the position of multiplicity, especially as propounded by Watkins, it seems almost inconceivable that another contradictory position could be argued with any credibility. But when confronted with the argument for antisocial personality, I feel almost equally convinced, even while keeping in mind the former. And each position was given about as competent, thorough, and well credentialed an endorsement by a mental health professional as is possible. When this occurs, I must ask myself another question. Is it possible that the two positions are *both right*? Is it either-*and*, rather than either-*or*? Or are both right, but only part of the story? If so, how can we reconcile the apparently irreconcilable?

At least *part* of Bianchi was antisocial in its most blatant form, that part-self going by the name of Steve, and to a lesser extent Billy as well. Neither part was in itself psychotic, but neither was under adequate awareness and control by Ken, accepting the dissociative position. Yet they were created by Ken, which raises the question of to what extent the creator is responsible for the creation. And close scrutiny of the accused's life history does show episodic antisocial behavior, whether or not this was done within the awareness or domain of any particular single ego state. Kenneth *as a whole* — a collective — certainly proved to have enough of the antisocial within him to justify the most extreme sanctions being applied by the court, if for no reason other than protection of society. None of the experts disputed this, to my knowledge. And that collection of experiences and feelings and behaviors known as "Steve" was *so* malevolent and destructive that it is hard to imagine Bianchi's being able to hold a job or a wife for even a short period of time without somehow setting this cauldron of fury aside, or decommissioning it — dissociation being the mode *par excellence*. So some dissociation with amnesia was extremely plausible; it is hard to conceive his functioning as his life history shows he did without some such "protective" device. Each position is true, then, but only part of the story. It becomes misleading only when one believes that the other position is excluded.

Achieving a hypnotic arm rigidity by voluntary choice also shows how fine the line is between voluntary and involuntary. Purposely making the arm stiff and rigid can become a hypnotic response when the experience and awareness of the choice slips beyond the awareness of he who is in charge (Appendix I). The subject who actually chose to tighten his arm at least fleetingly experienced it as just happening. There is at least one clear example in my own psychiatric practice of

where voluntary deception (conning) alternated with a true dissociated state. A dual personality to begin with, she at all times willfully
withheld information of undesirable behaviors from me to avoid disapproval, even while remaining in her primary ego state. At times this
process slipped beyond control, with subsequent amnesia, and without shifting into her other well defined alter-personality. Conscious
deception becomes major dissociation whenever that occurs, with the
typical amnesia. We temporarily have a new alter-personality. This
behavior then alternates between willful lying and true dissociation,
from the perspective of that ego state. Within that primary ego state
she alternated between duality and fusion. This case exemplifies how
close one is to the other, and I suspect this is much more common in
human life than recognized by our profession.

Carrying polar opposite positions to their ultimate conclusions (at
times absurdity) is commonplace in Anglo-American law. The adversary system itself assures this, since the system is designed to maximize
the likelihood that all the relevant information will be brought before
the court. A similar process is by no means unheard of within the
mental health profession, however, even with no legal stakes present.
We hear similar and equally irreconcilable arguments between two
psychiatrists about a given patient's diagnosis whenever that patient
rests in the "grey area" between the limits of relevance of two differently defined psychiatric syndromes. Is an agitated psychotic patient
schizophrenic, or is he manic? Those who fit the classic criteria present
no problem, but not all patients do.

Sometimes the most relevant diagnosis can be revealed only after a
long period of trial and error, most useful when we are continually
keeping our minds open for alternative explanations which can suggest alternative modes of problem-solving. I hope the present case
discussion will so highlight the necessity of a flexible either-and position. Even when a patient's diagnosis or formulation seems "obvious,"
another position might be equally justifiable. Which will work better,
or some combination of both, or an alternative altogether, may be resolvable in practice only by the test of time.

Some atypical patients subsequently prove to have dissociative disorder, and suddenly everything makes sense. But there are atypical
dissociators as well, and the same problem occurs with multiple personality as with any other psychiatric category. Precision and certain

ty are not there just because we would like them to be, no matter how neat and crisp our definitions. The psychiatrist must learn to live with psychic uncertainty — with simultaneous presence of paradoxes and polarities — if he is to maximize his flexibility and effectiveness.

Criminal Insanity

The Bianchi case highlights the absurdity of the "not guilty by reason of insanity" plea. The most pressing problem is this: If we grant that the most appropriate clinical diagnosis is multiple personality, then it would be necessary for the less appropriate diagnosis to be made for the most appropriate disposition. If multiple personality were to stick in court, there would be just too much risk that he would be "not guilty," and could presumably be set loose at some time at the discretion of some psychiatrist. And how could Kenneth Bianchi be *not* guilty, by any stretch of the imagination, at the simple commonsense level? If the person on trial is defined as the *whole* person or the orchestra within his head, no matter how split up, he must be guilty on the basis of the criminal evidence. Since human life as well as traditional psychiatry generally follows the whole person model fitting most people's experience, that is how the determination should go. Multiple consciousness does not clash with cohesive selfhood, but simply shows that we do not understand its essence as much as we would like, and that many levels contribute to this self.

To try Ken, Steve or Billy as if they each had separate bodies would be to commit the category error of defining as physically separate that which is just a sector of one personality which *experiences* itself as *like* a separate "self," and which is isolated from but yet must intersect with other levels of the overall Self. Yet this is exactly what the insanity "defense" attempts. *Ken* is not guilty because the offenses were committed by Steve, who was beyond Ken's awareness or control. Such a defense could be attempted logically only if one were to assume that part-selves are actually separate real Selves. But even if we assume (as I do *not*) that more than one soul inhabitated the body, then *each* must be tried. *Steve would* be guilty. Since punishment would involve incarceration of Steve's body, it must also involve that of Ken's, since the two are one and the same.

Not only would the "not guilty" plea require an assumption of multiplicity at a level which even I cannot accept, but it would also be logical only if one "personality" and not others were eligible for trial. If only the "president of the body" could be culpable, and one were to agree that Ken was the only *legitimate* "president," then one could argue not guilty. What is represented by Steve and Billy could be like subversive terrorists, and one might claim that what is done by terrorists would not be the responsibility of the nation at large. But Steve openly claimed right to the presidency of Bianchi's body, saying that he "deserved" it more. And he acted in that capacity while doing the rape-murders. I do not know of any rules of procedure for determining whose claim to the executive position is more legitimate in the family of Self comprising a single human individual.

Even if Ken (as a part-self) is the only one who can stand trial and be found culpable, we must then question to what extent Ken is responsible for Steve's actions. If subversive factions within a given nation cause gross damage to another nation, this might not have been the wish or intent of the first nation's leaders, but that nation might still have to assume responsibility and make restitution to the other. Since Ken created Steve, he is also responsible for him at least at the primary level.

All of these issues could be avoided if we make guilt and psychiatric status separate issues. An accused would be guilty or not guilty only on the basis of criminal evidence. If an individual's body committed a major offense, he is guilty whatever physical or mental condition might have caused his behavior. This is just simple commonsense logic. It in no way negates the more positive functions of the insanity plea, which had been instituted as a humanitarian means of showing compassion to one who truly committed a crime because of factors beyond control, who truly deserved compassion more than punishment. But a finding of guilty says nothing about how we must treat him, and does not prevent us from being compassionate towards him when indicated. It simply keeps the categories clear.

Determination of mental status could then be done as an entirely separate issue from whose body committed the offense. If insanity were found to be a mitigating factor, the complete verdict would be "*guilty*—by reason of insanity," which would carry different consequences than guilty and sane, but still define responsibility for the offense where it logically belongs.

Separation of guilt and mental status is desirable psychotherapeutically as well as legally. Not equivocating about guilt reinforces the fact that value judgments are appropriate primarily to behaviors, and helps to neutralize the category error so many patients make of putting their judgments against their basic being while letting go of control over the behaviors to which these value judgments more properly apply. When mental status is an entirely separate determination to be made on its own merits, without any bearing on legal guilt, it is much more likely that the examiner will be objective and compassionate, providing more validation of the patient's basic being. OKness of basic being is also reinforced, as well as responsibility for actions. With one simple readjustment of legal definitions, the law now becomes psychotherapeutic as well as more protective and effective.

Evaluator Variable, Resonance

Several individuals who observed the taped interviews of the accused, especially those by Watkins and Orne, noted that Bianchi's behavior was different with one than it was with the other. Even when shifting from one alter-personality to another this difference persisted, a difference hard to pinpoint in clear specific terms but which was easily sensed and seemed striking. With Watkins, he seemed genuine in all of the different ego states which emerged. This was compatible with this investigator's near certainty that the accused was, indeed, a true multiple personality. With Orne, however, there was a profound but intangible artificial quality. He seemed guarded and "unreal," and manifested that "caricatured" appearance whatever ego state he was in, which Orne used as evidence that he was willfully malingering. This different quality couldn't be attributed to dissociation since it presented across the board through all of the identified ego states. It appeared to one colleague that he was "giving each evaluator what he expected, or perhaps at least covertly wanted." If that is the case, what conclusions might we draw from that singular fact alone?

The first answer that comes to mind is psychopathy. Characteristic of the antisocial personality or psychopath is that he will deliberately behave in a way he believes will please his interrogator and serve his own ends, usually to such an unreal extent that he gives himself away to objective observers. Is Bianchi simply so much more skilled at this that he can fool the majority of experts? This would be the position taken by the prosecution.

Another possibility, worth careful attention because of its vast implications to the mental health profession, is the concept of *resonance* as set forth by Watkins (1978). This position assumes multiplicity in everyday life, that concurrent with one individual's verbal transactions, his multiple latent or "unconscious" ego states are also making themselves known loud and clear through nonverbal behavior. Similar latent ego states in the other individual are receiving these communications and responding to them in their own unique way, leading to other nonverbal communications. The social transactions are only the tip of the iceberg of what is actually going on. Ego states are so manifold, and nonverbal communication so rich at so many levels, that it would be unreasonable to expect that either party's responses could be entirely under voluntary control. A "therapeutic personality" is one whose latent ego states are able to validate latent ego states in another person and achieve a comfortable rapport, even without overt social communication. We feel comfortable and "at ease" with such a person, often highly trusting without really knowing why we should be so trusting. Without this resonance we are often likely to feel "on guard," even without fully knowing why. In turn, we behave "genuinely" to the former and defensively to the latter.

To explore the ramifications of the resonance concept to the Bianchi case we must attempt some "mind reading." We must come to a considered guess as to what covert nonverbal messages were being given out by the different evaluators, and responded to differently by the accused. First, Watkins was contracted by the defense and Orne by the prosecution. Even assuming, as I do, that each made maximal voluntary attempt to be objective, it would not be human for the above not to have at least some influence on evaluator behavior at some level. But a much more deeply seated bias could be inferred for each of the two from what is public knowledge about each—their different backgrounds, areas of expertise, and publicly stated views on significant issues.

Watkins is a leading expert on multiple personality, and is known as believing in the importance of multiple consciousness in everyday life. Even within this subspecialty, he is also close to the extreme position (shared by myself) that it works out best whenever possible to look for the OKness in even the most negative of selves and part-selves, and to utilize this. Like myself, he would attempt to "get rid of a persecutor" in only the most extreme of circumstances.

Orne, sharing a comparable expertise in hypnosis, has devoted

most of his life to research attempting to differentiate truly hypnotized subjects from simulators. He has found time and time again that
a skilled simulator can deceive even the most experienced of hypnotists, including himself, and has been studying how the distinction between hypnosis and simulation can be made with ever greater reliability. In addition, he has a long experience in forensic psychiatry. He
has been called to evaluate many criminal suspects, where there
would be all the reason in the world for the subject to want to deceive
the investigator.

Knowing only this, we could infer that Watkins would be likely to
convey the covert assumption at almost all levels that any person or
part-person is OK in its basic being. Even when one commits the most
reprehensible of behavioral offenses, if we look hard enough we can
explain it as, at the very worst, a gross perversion of what is the otherwise positive life instinct. This would facilitate the subject's talking
openly, appearing more "real." Orne would more likely convey a certain suspiciousness, a covert belief rooted in and substantiated by
years of experience, that one can never take a subject's communications at face value, one should always look for willful deception, especially when the motivation for this is as pressing as being faced with a
major felony charge.

Taking the above assumptions, I would predict that the accused
would sense a positive bias in Watkins' presence which extends to
multiple and very deep levels. He and all his latent ego states would be
more likely to feel safe, and to want to share their experience as they in
fact experience it. The communications would come across as more
congruent, then, and more genuine or "real." Responding to Orne,
however, he would sense that virtually everything he said would be
subject to critical scrutiny, and knowing that the evidence of the case
assures his actual guilt, he would certainly feel terribly on guard.
Knowing the stakes, he would almost certainly want to pick and
choose most carefully what he said to the investigator, and this defensiveness would extend throughout nearly his entire being. The result
could easily be that "unreal" or "caricatured" quality which Orne correctly cited. What is ironic is that this would convince each investigator that the original covert assumptions were indeed accurate.
Whether or not the accused was truly hypnotized or was simulating
might even have varied from investigator to investigator. He might

have been truly hypnotized for Watkins and simulating for Orne as a result of the different communications he was receiving from each.

If we take literally the observation that he was more "genuine" with Watkins than with Orne, one might take that as evidence that the former's position was more plausible. So now we are again in a situation where we can use the different behavior as an argument for either position — multiple or psychopath, tragic victim of a disordered life or a willful evildoer. Again, I doubt that it must be either-or.

This puts into relief a "criticism" frequently leveled at multiplicity by the psychiatric community at large, that a "multiple personality" is often an iatrogenic reponse of a patient to a physician who has special interest in this area. Do many patients whom Watkins or I would diagnosis as multiples behave in order to satisfy *our* expectations or covert wishes? If evaluator variables can have so profound an effect on diagnosis as the above suggests, what is the role of *artifact* in the diagnosis of multiple personality? Reviewing Watkins' arguments, one can see that there might be implied suggestion occurring at several points, especially point (c) where "Steve" was first called forth. But artifact works both ways. The inadvertently introduced therapeutic suggestion (d) which followed might have led to an eroding of the dissociative barrier which would affect subsequent evaluations. And Orne's evaluation was indeed subsequent.

Communication of a psychiatrist's beliefs and expectations through his behavior no doubt occurs, and a patient will unavoidably respond differently with different communications of his own, and these cannot help but influence the psychiatrist's diagnostic impressions. Even if multiple personality and its equivalents gain greater acceptance within psychiatry, I would still not be surprised if I would make the diagnosis more frequently than one who looks askance upon this area of inquiry. But I cannot create a multiple personality where there is nothing corresponding to the diagnosis. Where this type of artifact might occur is at the limits of relevance of a diagnostic category or concept. It is only when the patient is in the grey area between multiple personality and some other category that my personality will influence his behavior more towards the former position.

This phenomenon is not limited to the diagnosis of multiple personality. Biologically oriented psychiatrists are most likely to see a depressive state as endogenous, and they will get far better results with pharmacological treatment than a more psychodynamically oriented therapist, even in the same patient. Some psychiatrists diagnose more patients as schizophrenic; others more patients as manic. The first are more likely to be successful in use of antipsychotic drugs, the latter more effective with lithium — even for the same patient, if that patient fits within the border between the two.

Relativity of diagnosis and treatment to the bias of a given psychiatrist, legendary in our profession, does not necessarily expose a great inadequacy of this profession, but contributes to our understanding of its nature. The A/Not-A Absurdity or psychic uncertainty appears again, and cannot be avoided. But I cannot see the fact that more than one seemingly contradictory position can be true, and that more than one treatment modality might work, as necessarily a flaw. At another level, it is a reflection of the marvelous adaptability of the human organism. Multilevel functioning may be one of the more striking features of this adaptability, still so far beyond our total understanding.

References

Allison, R. B., A New Treatment Approach for Multiple Personalities. *American Journal of Clinical Hypnosis*, 1974, 17, 15-32.

_____. Psychotherapy of Multiple Personality, 1977, unpublished monograph.

_____. A Rational Psychotherapy Plan for Multiplicity, *Svensk Tidskrift for Hypnos*, 1978, Nr 3-4, 9-16.

_____. Personal Communication, 1979.

American Psychiatric Association. *Diagnostic and Statistical Manual of Psychiatric Disorders. III.* Washington, D.C.: APA, 1980.

Arieti, S. *Creativity, the Magic Synthesis*. New York, Basic Books, Inc., 1976.

Bandler, B. and Grinder, J. *The Structure of Magic, I and II,* Palo Alto, CA., Science and Behavior Books, 1975.

Barber, T. X., An Alternative Paradigm. In: Fromm, E. and Shor, R. E. (eds.), *Hypnosis: Research Developments and Perspectives.* Chicago/New York, Aldine-Atherton, 1972, 115-182.

_____. Personal Communication, 1975.

_____. Personal Communication, 1977.

Beahrs, J. O., The Hypnotic Psychotherapy of Milton H. Erickson. *American Journal of Clinical Hypnosis,* 1971, 14, 73-90.

_____. *That Which Is: An Inquiry into the Nature of Energy, Ethics, and Mental Health.* Portland, OR., Integrated Arts, Inc., orig. 1977(a).

_____. Integrating Erickson's Approach, *American Journal of Clinical Hypnosis,* 1977, 20, 55-68(b).

_____. Cure: An Opportunity for Yes-Butting. *Transactional Analysis Journal,* 1980, 10, 131-132.

_____. Understanding Erickson's Approach. In: Zeig, J. K. (ed.) *Ericksonian Approaches to Hypnosis and Psychotherapy.* New York, Brunner/Mazel, 1982.

223

Beahrs, J. O. and Humiston, K. E., Dynamics of Experiential Therapy, *American Journal of Clinical Hypnosis*, 1974, 17, 1-14.

Berne, Eric. *Transactional Analysis in Psychotherapy*. New York, Grove Press, 1961.

_____. *Principles of Group Treatment*. New York, Oxford Univ. Press, 1966.

_____. *What Do You Say After You Say Hello?* New York, Grove Press, 1972.

Bernheim, H. *Suggestive Therapeutics* (1890), New York, London Book Co., 1947.

Bleuler, E. *Dementia Praecox, or the Group of Schizophrenias* (1911). New York, International Universities Press, 1952.

Bohm, D., Quantum Theory as an Indication of a New Order in Physics. Part A. The Development of New Orders as Shown Through the History of Physics, *Foundations of Physics*, 1971, 1, 359-381.

Bohr, Niels. *Atomic Physics and Human Knowledge*. New York, Science Editions, Inc. 1961.

Braun, B. G., Personal Communication, 1979.

_____. Hypnosis for Multiple Personalities. In: H. J. Wain (ed.), *Clinical Hypnosis in Medicine*, Chicago/London, Yearbook Medical Publishers, 1980, pp. 209-217.

Brill, Earl H. *The Christian Moral Vision*. New York, The Seabury Press, 1979, p. 43.

Calof, David, Personal Communication, 1979.

Congden, M. H., Hain, J., and Stevenson, I., A Case of Multiple Personality Illustrating the Transition from Role Playing, *Journal of Nervous and Mental Diseases*, 1965, 13, 497.

Donington, R. *Wagner's "Ring" and Its Symbols*. London, Faber & Faber, 1963.

Edmonston, W. E., Relaxation as an Appropriate Experimental Control in Hypnosis, *American Journal of Clinical Hypnosis*, 1972, 14, 218-229.

English, Fanita, What Shall I Do Tomorrow?: Reconceptualizing Transactional Analysis. In: Barnes, G. (ed.), *Transactional Analysis After Eric Berne*. New York, Harper and Row, 1977, 287-347.

Erickson, M. H., Personal Communication, 1972.

_____. Personal Communication, 1976.

Erickson, M. H. and Rossi, E. L. *Hypnotherapy: An Exploratory Casebook*. New York, Irvington Publishers, Inc., 1979.

Esdaile, James. *Hypnosis in Medicine and Surgery* (1846). New York, Julian Press, Inc., 1957.

Federn, Paul. *Ego Psychology and the Psychoses*. (E. Weiss, Ed.), New York, Basic Books, 1952.

Feynman, R. P., Leighton, R. B., and Sands, M. *The Feynman Lectures on Physics*. Menlo Park, CA., Addison-Wesley, 1963.

Flavell, John. *The Developmental Psychology of Jean Piaget*. New York, Van Nostrand Co., 1963.

Frankel, F. H. *Hypnosis: Trance as a Coping Mechanism*. New York/London, Plenum Medical Book Co., 1976.

Freud, S. *The Interpretation of Dreams* (1900). New York, Avon, 1965.

_____. *Introductory Lectures of Psychoanalysis* (1916). New York, Doubleday, 1943.

_____. *Group Psychology and Analysis of the Ego* (1920). New York, Norton, 1975.

_____. *New Introductory Lectures on Psychoanalysis*. New York, Norton, 1933.

Fromm, E. *The Anatomy of Human Destructiveness.* New York, Holt, Rinehart and Winston, 1973.

Gallwey, W. T. *The Inner Game of Tennis.* New York, Random House, 1974.

————. *Inner Tennis: Playing the Game.* New York, Random House, 1976.

Gill, M. M. and Brenman, M. *Hypnosis and Related States: Psychoanalytic Studies in Regression.* New York, International Universities Press, 1959.

Grinker, R. R., Sr. The Relevance of General Systems Theory to Psychiatry. In: Arieti, S. (ed.), *American Handbook of Psychiatry,* Vol. VI, 251–271. New York, Basic Books, 1975.

Gruenewald, D., Multiple Personality and Splitting Phenomena: A Reconceptualization, *Journal of Nervous and Mental Diseases,* 1977, 164, 385.

Haley, Jay. *Strategies of Psychotherapy.* New York, Grune and Stratton, 1963.

Harriman, P. L., A New Approach to Multiple Personalities, *American Journal of Orthopsychiatry,* 1943, 13, 636.

Hawksworth, H. and Schwarz, T. *The Five of Me.* Chicago, Henry Regnery Co., 1977.

Hebb, D. O. *Organization of Behavior.* New York, Wiley, 1949.

Hilgard, E. R. *The Experience of Hypnosis: A Shorter Version of Hypnotic Susceptibility.* New York, Harcourt, Brace & World, Inc., 1968.

————. *Divided Consciousness: Multiple Controls in Human Thought and Action.* New York, John Wiley and Sons, 1977.

Hilgard, E. R. and Hilgard, J. R., *Hypnosis in the Relief of Pain.* Los Altos, CA., William Kaufman, Inc., 1975.

Hilgard, J. R. *Personality and Hypnosis: A Study of Imaginative Involvement.* Chicago, University of Chicago Press, 1970.

Horowitz, M. J., Pathological Grief and the Activation of Latent Self-Images, *American Journal of Psychiatry,* 1980, 137, 1157–1162.

Humiston, K. E., Personal Communication, 1976.

James, W. *Principles of Psychology.* New York, Dover, 1890.

————. *The Varieties of Religious Experience* (1902). New York, Macmillan, 1961.

Jung, C. G. *Man and His Symbols.* London, Aldus Books, 1964.

Kampman, R., Hypnotically Induced Multiple Personality: An Experimental Study, *International Journal of Clinical and Experimental Hypnosis,* 1976, 24, 215–227.

Karpman, S. B., Fairy Tales and Script Drama Analysis, *Transactional Analysis Bulletin,* 1968, 7, 39–43.

Kernberg, O. *Borderline Conditions and Pathological Narcissism.* New York, Jason Aronson, 1975.

Kline, Milton V. Freud and Hypnosis: A Re-evaluation, *Journal of Clinical and Experimental Hypnosis,* 1972, 20 (4), 252–263.

Kohut, H., Forms and Transformations of Narcissism, *Journal of the American Psychoanalytic Association,* 1966, 14, 243–272.

————. *The Analysis of the Self.* New York, International Universities Press, 1971.

————. *The Restoration of the Self.* New York, International Universities Press, 1977.

LeCron, L. *Self-Hypnotism: The Technique and Its Use in Daily Living* (1964). New York, Signet, 1970.

Lowen, A. *The Betrayal of the Body.* New York, Macmillan, 1967.

_____. *Depression and the Body*. New York, Coward, McCann, and Geoghegan, 1972.

_____. *Bioenergetics*. New York, Coward, McCann, and Geoghegan, 1975.

Lundeholm, H., An Experimental Study of Functional Anesthesia Induced by Suggestion in Hypnosis, *Journal of Abnormal and Social Psychology*, 1928, 23, 337-355.

Martin, P. A., Dynamic Considerations of the Hysterical Psychosis, *American Journal of Psychiatry*, 1971, 128, 745-748.

May, P. R. A. *Treatment of Schizophrenia: A Comparative Study of Five Treatment Methods*. New York, Science House, 1968.

Orne, M. T., The Nature of Hypnosis: Artifact and Essence, *Journal of Abnormal and Social Psychology*, 1959, 58, 277-299.

Perls, F. S. *Gestalt Therapy Verbatim*. Lafayette, CA., Real People Press, 1969.

Pines, Maya, Invisible Playmates, *Psychology Today*, May 1978, 11, 23.

Prince, M. *The Dissociation of a Personality* (1906). New York, Greenwood Press, 1969.

Roberts, Jane. *The Coming of Seth*. New York: Pocket Books, 1976. A reprinting of *How To Develop Your ESP Power*. New York: Frederick Fell, 1966.

_____. *Seth Speaks: The Eternal Validity of the Soul*. Englewood Cliffs, N.J., Prentice Hall, Inc. 1972.

_____. *The Nature of Personal Reality: A Seth Book*. Englewood Cliffs, N.J., Prentice hall, Inc., 1974.

_____. *Psychic Politics: An Aspect Psychology Book*. Englewood Cliffs, N.J., Prentice Hall, Inc., 1976.

_____. *The Afterdeath Journal of an American Philosopher: The World View of William James*. Englewood Cliffs, N.J., Prentice Hall, Inc., 1978.

Sarbin, T. R. and Coe, W. C. *Hypnosis: A Social Psychological Analysis of Influence Communication*. New York, Holt, Rinehart and Winston, 1972.

Sheehan, P. W. and Perry, C. W. *Methodologies of Hypnosis: A Critical Appraisal of Contemporary Paradigms of Hypnosis*. Hillsdale, N.J., Lawrence Erlbaum Associates, 1976.

Sizemore, C. C. *I'm Eve*. New York, Jove Publications, 1977.

Spinoza, B. *The Ethics* (1677). New York, Dover, 1951.

Steiner, C. *Games Alcoholics Play*. New York,Grove Press, 1971.

_____. The Pig Parent, *Transactional Analysis Journal*, 1979, 9, 26-40.

Stern, Charles. *The Etiology of Identity Splitting in Multiple Personality Dissociations*. Ann Arbor: Universities Microfilms International, 1980.

Sullivan, H. S. *The Interpersonal Theory of Psychiatry*. New York, Norton, 1953.

Tart, C. T. *States of Consciousness*. New York, E. P. Dutton & Co., 1975.

Teller, E. *The Pursuit of Simplicity*. Malibu, CA., Pepperdine University Press, 1980.

Tillich, P. *Systematic Theology*, Vol. I. Chicago, University of Chicago Press, 1951.

Watkins, J. G. *The Therapeutic Self*. New York, Human Sciences Press, 1978.

_____. Personal Communication, 1979.

Watkins, H. H. *The Woman in Black and the Lady in White*. New York, Norton, 1980.

Watkins, J. G. and Watkins, H. H., Ego States and Hidden Observers, *Journal of Altered States of Consciousness*, 1979-80, 5 (1979a).

_____ & _____. The Theory and Practice of Ego State Therapy. In: Grayson, H. (ed). *Short-Term Approaches to Psychotherapy*. New York, National Institute for the Psychotherapies and Human Sciences Press, 1979(b).

_____ & _____. Personal Communication, 1980.

Watzlawick, P. *How Real is Real?* New York, Random House, 1976.

Watzlawick, P., Weakland, J., and Fisch, R. *Change: Principles of Problem Formation and Problem Resolution.* New York, Norton, 1974.

Weitzenhoffer, A. M., and Hilgard, E. R. *Stanford Hypnotic Susceptibility Scales, Forms A and B.* Palo Alto, Consulting Psychologists Press, 1959.

Index